Statistical Methods for Overdispersed Count Data

In memory of my father

To my daughter, Laura

Biostatistics and Health Science Set

coordinated by
Mounir Mesbah

Statistical Methods for Overdispersed Count Data

Jean-François Dupuy

ELSEVIER

First published 2018 in Great Britain and the United States by ISTE Press Ltd and Elsevier Ltd

ISTE Press Ltd
27-37 St George's Road
London SW19 4EU
UK

www.iste.co.uk

Elsevier Ltd
The Boulevard, Langford Lane
Kidlington, Oxford, OX5 1GB
UK

www.elsevier.com

Notices
Knowledge and best practice in this field are constantly changing. As new research and experience broaden our understanding, changes in research methods, professional practices, or medical treatment may become necessary.

Practitioners and researchers must always rely on their own experience and knowledge in evaluating and using any information, methods, compounds, or experiments described herein. In using such information or methods they should be mindful of their own safety and the safety of others, including parties for whom they have a professional responsibility.

To the fullest extent of the law, neither the Publisher nor the authors, contributors, or editors, assume any liability for any injury and/or damage to persons or property as a matter of products liability, negligence or otherwise, or from any use or operation of any methods, products, instructions, or ideas contained in the material herein.

For information on all our publications visit our website at http://store.elsevier.com/

British Library Cataloguing-in-Publication Data
A CIP record for this book is available from the British Library
Library of Congress Cataloging in Publication Data
A catalog record for this book is available from the Library of Congress
ISBN 978-1-78548-266-3

Printed and bound in the UK and US

Contents

Introduction

This book describes statistical methods for analyzing overdispersed count data. Data are said to be overdispersed if the variance of the observations is greater than the variance predicted by the theoretical model. This can be due to various reasons. To provide just a few examples, if key explanatory variables were omitted from the model, if outliers are present among the observations or if there is an unobserved heterogeneity between the individuals in the sample, then overdispersion can arise as a result.

Another major cause of overdispersion is an excessive number of observations equal to zero (described as an "excess of zeros" or "zero inflation"). This can happen in fields ranging from the most "classical" applications – insurance (especially automotive insurance, with the no-claims bonus/penalty system), economics (e.g. in healthcare, when studying healthcare consumption and the factors determining non-continuation of medical care), epidemiology and sociology (the factors that prompt individuals to leave their social benefits unclaimed) – to the most unexpected of places, such as conflict analysis and terrorism.

Although the first statistical models for zero-inflated count data were developed in the 1960s, sophisticated models did not truly begin to take form until the early 2000s. Nevertheless, there are three precursory milestones that need to be mentioned: Mullahy [MUL 86], Lambert [LAM 92] and Hall [HAL 00]. These authors proposed the first *regression-based* zero-inflated models, laying the foundations of the methodological, theoretical and applied research that would follow.

The objective of regression is to model and study the relationship between one variable (response variable) and one or several others (explanatory variables). Linear regression models are the mostly widely studied topic of regression, followed by classical count models (binomial and Poisson regression models, to mention the two most common ones). These models are often presented within the unified framework of generalized linear models, which were introduced by Nelder and Wedderburn [NEL 72]. At present, they are taught in every course on statistical engineering, econometrics, biostatistics and so on; more generally, they are still a crucial part of any university course that touches upon statistical modeling. By contrast, techniques designed to account for overdispersion (variance correction methods, zero-inflated models) are less widely studied.

This book aims to provide readers with an introduction to these methods, without attempting an exhaustive treatment – the subject is simply too vast to study! Much more modestly, we simply aim to present a few of the most classical tools for managing overdispersion in count data. Each tool is presented rigorously, but excessive formalism is avoided to ensure that the book remains accessible to any reader with a grasp of standard results from linear algebra and enough probability theory to understand statistical modeling. The more technical sections on the asymptotics of zero-inflated regression models can be safely omitted without detracting from the rest of the book.

Each tool and method described in this book is concretely illustrated by applications based on real data and processed using the open-source and freely available statistical software package R [RCO 17]. The same data set serves as a single guiding thread in Chapters 2–4. These data were collected by a national study on medical spending in the United States and are directly included in the AER package [KLE 08] of R. Our specific objective is to illustrate the methods and statistical models that can be used to account for overdispersion. Accordingly, we did neither try to establish the finest possible explanatory model, for example, by looking for interactions between the explanatory variables, nor attempt to validate the models used as illustrations in this book. Readers interested in these aspects (use of residuals, influence measures, diagnostic tools, etc.) are very welcome to explore some of the (many!) other more specialized publications on these topics.

Zero-inflated regression models will occupy a large portion of this book. Chapter 4 is exclusively dedicated to these models. An understanding of some of the basic notions of generalized linear models (model formalism, construction of estimators and tests, numerical aspects) is required before reading this chapter. The best way to acquire a clear understanding of these notions is to start from scratch with linear regression. This book is therefore organized as follows. Chapter 1 gives an introduction to linear regression models, followed by Chapter 2, which presents generalized linear models, with special emphasis on binomial and Poisson regression models. Chapter 3 introduces the subject of overdispersed count data and outlines a few statistical tools and models that can be used to account for overdispersion. Chapter 4 tackles the more specific question of zero-inflated regression models. Much of this chapter is dedicated to reviewing recent work in this field. In particular, we examine the question of identifiability for this type of model and explore its practical ramifications for model construction. We also discuss the asymptotic properties of the maximum likelihood estimator for these models. Although this section of the book is more theoretical and undoubtedly makes for drier reading, its importance should not be underestimated by practitioners of statistics. The applicability of standard statistical inference techniques based on asymptotic arguments, such as those used in generalized linear models, is justified here.

1

A Brief Overview of Linear Models

Generalized linear regression models are the global framework of this book, but we shall only introduce them in Chapter 2. Chapter 1 is dedicated to (standard and Gaussian) linear regression models. Despite just being a special case of generalized linear models, linear models need to be discussed separately for a few reasons. Performing linear regression in a Gaussian setting always leads to specific distributions (e.g. for the test statistics), regardless of sample size. By contrast, when working with generalized linear models, test statistics and confidence intervals are constructed by asymptotic arguments. Furthermore, generalized linear models are an extremely general approach to expressing the relationship between a response variable and a set of explanatory variables. It is easier to appreciate the benefits of these tools by considering the special case of Gaussian linear models before introducing the general formalism.

1.1. Introduction

In general terms, a regression model allows us to formulate the relation between a variable Z, known as the explained variable (response variable, endogenous variable or dependent variable), and a set of explanatory variables $X_1, X_2, \ldots, X_p$, also known as the covariables, regressors, exogenous variables or independent variables.

To construct a regression model of Z in terms of $X_1, X_2, \ldots, X_p$ means to find a function f such that $f(X_1, X_2, \ldots, X_p)$ gives the best possible approximation of Z. Our purpose in doing so can vary. For example, we may wish to find a relation between Z and $X_1, X_2, \ldots, X_p$ in order to understand and interpret a phenomenon (this type of problem is very common in a wide variety of fields such as biology, economics, physics and sociology). Alternatively, given a set of explanatory variables, we may wish to distinguish the variables that significantly affect the response from those that do not. Similarly, we might want to evaluate ("*estimate*") the effect of each regressor on the variable Z. In the context of a modeling problem, we could even use the model obtained by regression to predict the value of Z for arbitrary values of $X_1, X_2, \ldots, X_p$.

In statistics, these objectives are accomplished by collecting observations about individuals (an individual in the statistical sense is not necessarily a physical person). In the context of regression, each individual observation takes the form of a pair:

$$(Z_i, \mathbf{X}_i), \quad i = 1, \ldots, n,$$

where Z_i denotes the response variable observed at the i-th individual and $\mathbf{X}_i$ is the set of explanatory variables $(X_{i1}, \ldots, X_{ip})$ measured at this individual. Together, the pairs $\{(Z_1, \mathbf{X}_1), \ldots, (Z_n, \mathbf{X}_n)\}$ make up the observation sample, which has size n. It is assumed that n is larger than p.

The linear model is the most widely known regression model and the first encountered by students. This model assumes that there is an affine relation between Z and $X_1, X_2, \ldots, X_p$ (often called a linear relation, by abuse of terminology). The Gaussian linear model is a special case of a generalized linear model. It makes sense for us to begin by recalling a few ideas about this model. A good understanding of the tools of statistical inference used by this model will be useful later when we consider similar problems with other generalized linear models and zero-inflated models. However, our goal is not to give an exhaustive explanation of linear models in this chapter. Readers interested in studying them in more depth can refer to one of the many comprehensive publications dedicated to the subject. Even just the references would be impossible to list exhaustively. Four particularly noteworthy examples written in French are [ANT 92, AZA 06, COR 07, GUY 01]. Other references, including English publications, are easy to find.

1.2. The standard linear model

For $i = 1, \ldots, n$, the linear model can be stated as:

$$Z_i = \beta_1 + \beta_2 X_{i2} + \ldots + \beta_p X_{ip} + \epsilon_i$$
$$= \beta^\top \mathbf{X}_i + \epsilon_i, \qquad\qquad [1.1]$$

where $\top$ denotes the transpose of a vector (or matrix) and $\mathbf{X}_i$ denotes the column vector $\mathbf{X}_i = (X_{i1}, X_{i2}, \ldots, X_{ip})^\top \in \mathbb{R}^p$. The real number $\beta^\top \mathbf{X}_i$ is called the linear predictor. The column vector $\beta = (\beta_1, \ldots, \beta_p)^\top$ in $\mathbb{R}^p$ is called a model parameter, regression parameter or regression coefficient. This is an unknown parameter; to accomplish the objectives stated in the Introduction, we need to estimate this parameter from the observations $(Z_i, \mathbf{X}_i), i = 1, \ldots, n$. The process of estimating β is described as fitting the model (to the data). The term ϵ_i is an unknown noise term (an error term).

REMARK.– The model in equation [1.1] is usually parameterized in such a way that $X_{i1} = 1$. In this case, the parameter β_1 is called the (vertical) intercept, or the constant. The model

$$Z_i = \beta_1 + \beta_2 X_{i2} + \epsilon_i,$$

in a single explanatory variable (other than the constant term 1), is called a simple linear regression model. The more general model in equation [1.1] is known as a multiple linear regression model.   □

The term "linear" in "linear model" means that the model is linear in β. The following models are also linear models:

$$Z_i = \beta_1 + \beta_2 X_{i2}^2 + \epsilon_i \text{ and } Z_i = \beta_1 + \beta_2 X_{i2} + \beta_3 X_{i3} + \beta_4 X_{i2} X_{i3} + \epsilon_i.$$

The vector β of the model in equation [1.1] can be estimated by the method of least squares without making any assumptions about the distribution of the observations. This method is introduced in section 1.3. However, to construct confidence intervals and test statistics for the β_j, we need to formulate a hypothesis regarding the distribution of the ϵ_i (see section 1.4).

1.3. Least squares estimator

Let

$$
\mathbb{X} = \begin{pmatrix}
1 & X_{12} & \cdots & X_{1p} \\
1 & X_{22} & \cdots & X_{2p} \\
\vdots & \vdots & \ddots & \vdots \\
1 & X_{n2} & \cdots & X_{np}
\end{pmatrix}
$$

be the $n \times p$ matrix whose i-th row contains the values $\mathbf{X}_i^\top = (1, X_{i2}, \ldots, X_{ip})$ taken by the p explanatory variables at the i-th individual; in other words, the j-th column of this matrix contains the values $X_{1j}, \ldots, X_{nj}$ taken by the j-th explanatory variable at each of the n individuals in the sample. This matrix is known as the *design matrix*.

Furthermore, let $\mathbf{Z} = (Z_1, \ldots, Z_n)^\top \in \mathbb{R}^n$ be the column vector containing the n observations of the response variable, and let $\mathbf{E} = (\epsilon_1, \ldots, \epsilon_n)^\top \in \mathbb{R}^n$ be the column vector of n error terms. The model in equation [1.1] can be written in matrix form as follows:

$$
\mathbf{Z} = \mathbb{X}\beta + \mathbf{E}.
$$

We will assume that the matrix $\mathbb{X}$ is full rank (the advantage of this hypothesis $\mathcal{H}_1$ will become clear soon). If the number n of individuals is larger than the number p of explanatory variables, as we assumed earlier, then the rank of $\mathbb{X}$ is p. This is equivalent to assuming that the explanatory variables $X_1, X_2, \ldots, X_p$ are linearly independent.

REMARK.– If $\mathbb{X}$ is full rank, then it is easy to check that $\mathbb{X}^\top \mathbb{X}$ (which is a real symmetric $p \times p$ matrix) is invertible. Indeed, we can show that it is positive definite as follows (recall that a $p \times p$ real symmetric matrix is said to be positive definite if $u^\top M u > 0$ for every non-zero vector u in $\mathbb{R}^p$).

Let u be a non-zero vector in $\mathbb{R}^p$ and $\|u\|$ be the Euclidean norm of u. Then, $u^\top (\mathbb{X}^\top \mathbb{X}) u = \|\mathbb{X}u\|^2 \geq 0$. Suppose that $\|\mathbb{X}u\|^2 = 0$. Then, $\mathbb{X}u = 0$, and since $\mathbb{X}$ is assumed to have rank p, it follows that $u = 0$, which is a contradiction, so the inequality $u^\top (\mathbb{X}^\top \mathbb{X}) u > 0$ necessarily holds. The matrix $\mathbb{X}^\top \mathbb{X}$ is therefore positive definite and hence invertible. $\square$

The least squares estimator $\hat{\beta}$ of β is defined as the value that minimizes the residual sum of squares (RSS):

$$RSS(\beta) = \sum_{i=1}^{n} \left(Z_i - \beta^{\top} \mathbf{X}_i \right)^2$$

$$= (\mathbf{Z} - \mathbb{X}\beta)^{\top} (\mathbf{Z} - \mathbb{X}\beta)$$

$$= \|\mathbf{Z} - \mathbb{X}\beta\|^2.$$

Notationally, we write:

$$\hat{\beta} = \arg\min_{\beta \in \mathbb{R}^p} \|\mathbf{Z} - \mathbb{X}\beta\|^2.$$

There are several ways to find an expression for $\hat{\beta}$. Its value is fixed by the following theorem:

THEOREM.– If the matrix $\mathbb{X}$ is full rank, then the least squares estimator $\hat{\beta}$ of β is:

$$\hat{\beta} = \left(\mathbb{X}^{\top}\mathbb{X} \right)^{-1} \mathbb{X}^{\top}\mathbf{Z}.$$

Expression of the least squares estimator: proof

One way of computing $\hat{\beta}$ is to differentiate the function

$$RSS(\beta) = \mathbf{Z}^{\top}\mathbf{Z} - \mathbf{Z}^{\top}\mathbb{X}\beta - \beta^{\top}\mathbb{X}^{\top}\mathbf{Z} + \beta^{\top}\mathbb{X}^{\top}\mathbb{X}\beta$$

$$= \mathbf{Z}^{\top}\mathbf{Z} - 2\mathbf{Z}^{\top}\mathbb{X}\beta + \beta^{\top}\mathbb{X}^{\top}\mathbb{X}\beta$$

with respect to β and then solve the equation $\left. \frac{\partial RSS(\beta)}{\partial \beta} \right|_{\beta=\hat{\beta}} = 0$. This gives:

$$\frac{\partial RSS(\beta)}{\partial \beta} = -2\mathbb{X}^{\top}\mathbf{Z} + 2\mathbb{X}^{\top}\mathbb{X}\beta,$$

and so $\hat{\beta}$ satisfies $\mathbb{X}^\top \mathbb{X} \hat{\beta} = \mathbb{X}^\top \mathbf{Z}$. We showed earlier that $\mathbb{X}^\top \mathbb{X}$ is invertible subject to the assumption that $\text{rank}(\mathbb{X}) = p$. We can therefore write that $\hat{\beta} = \left(\mathbb{X}^\top \mathbb{X}\right)^{-1} \mathbb{X}^\top \mathbf{Z}$.

We still need to verify that $\hat{\beta}$ is a minimum of $RSS(\beta)$. To do this, we can check that the $p \times p$ matrix of second partial derivatives of $RSS(\beta)$ is positive definite. The second derivatives have the expression:

$$\frac{\partial^2 RSS(\beta)}{\partial \beta \partial \beta^\top} = 2\mathbb{X}^\top \mathbb{X}.$$

We showed earlier that $\mathbb{X}^\top \mathbb{X}$ is positive definite (see the previous remark), so this completes the proof. $\qquad\square$

The least squares estimator can also be constructed and interpreted geometrically. Given a vector u in $\mathbb{R}^n$ and a vector subspace $\mathcal{S}$ of $\mathbb{R}^n$, we recall that the orthogonal projection of u onto $\mathcal{S}$ (denoted Pu) is defined as the vector of $\mathcal{S}$ that minimizes $\|u - v\|^2$ for $v \in \mathcal{S}$. In other words:

$$\|u - Pu\|^2 = \min_{v \in \mathcal{S}} \|u - v\|^2.$$

The set $\mathcal{S}_{\mathbb{X}} := \{\mathbb{X}\beta : \beta \in \mathbb{R}^p\}$ forms a vector subspace of $\mathbb{R}^n$ spanned by the column vectors of the matrix $\mathbb{X}$ (the dimension of $\mathcal{S}_{\mathbb{X}}$ is p because these columns are assumed to be linearly independent). Minimizing $RSS(\beta) = \|\mathbf{Z} - \mathbb{X}\beta\|^2$ with respect to β is therefore equivalent to finding the closest element of $\mathcal{S}_{\mathbb{X}}$ to $\mathbf{Z} \in \mathbb{R}^n$ with respect to the usual Euclidean norm. This element is defined as the orthogonal projection of $\mathbf{Z}$ onto $\mathcal{S}_{\mathbb{X}}$.

Writing P for the orthogonal projection mapping onto $\mathcal{S}_{\mathbb{X}}$ and I_n for the identity matrix of order n, the vector $\mathbf{Z} \in \mathbb{R}^n$ can be uniquely decomposed into the sum:

$$\mathbf{Z} = P\mathbf{Z} + (I_n - P)\mathbf{Z},$$

where $P\mathbf{Z}$ belongs to $\mathcal{S}_{\mathbb{X}}$ and $(I_n - P)\mathbf{Z}$ belongs to the orthogonal complement of $\mathcal{S}_{\mathbb{X}}$. The vector $(I_n - P)\mathbf{Z}$ is therefore orthogonal to every vector v in $\mathcal{S}_{\mathbb{X}}$.

But every vector in $\mathcal{S}_{\mathbb{X}}$ can be written in the form $\mathbb{X}\alpha$, for $\alpha \in \mathbb{R}^p$. Thus, for all $\alpha \in \mathbb{R}^p$, the scalar product $\langle \mathbb{X}\alpha, (I_n - P)\mathbf{Z} \rangle$ is zero. In other words:

$$0 = \langle \mathbb{X}\alpha, (I_n - P)\mathbf{Z} \rangle = \alpha^\top \mathbb{X}^\top (I_n - P)\mathbf{Z} = \alpha^\top (\mathbb{X}^\top \mathbf{Z} - \mathbb{X}^\top P\mathbf{Z}).$$

Since this relation holds for every $\alpha \in \mathbb{R}^p$, it follows that $\mathbb{X}^\top \mathbf{Z} = \mathbb{X}^\top P\mathbf{Z}$, where $P\mathbf{Z} = \mathbb{X}\hat{\beta}$. This gives $\hat{\beta} = \left(\mathbb{X}^\top \mathbb{X} \right)^{-1} \mathbb{X}^\top \mathbf{Z}$, as before.

REMARK.– We note that:

$$P\mathbf{Z} = \mathbb{X}\hat{\beta} = \mathbb{X} \left(\mathbb{X}^\top \mathbb{X} \right)^{-1} \mathbb{X}^\top \mathbf{Z},$$

which allows us to deduce an expression for the matrix of the orthogonal projection mapping onto the subspace generated by the columns of $\mathbb{X}$:

$$P = \mathbb{X} \left(\mathbb{X}^\top \mathbb{X} \right)^{-1} \mathbb{X}^\top.$$

It is straightforward to check that P satisfies the usual properties of an orthogonal projection mapping ($P^2 = P, P = P^\top$). This matrix is sometimes called the "hat matrix" H, inspired by the popular notation $\hat{\mathbf{Z}} := P\mathbf{Z}$. The matrix P sends $\mathbf{Z}$ to $\hat{\mathbf{Z}}$ (pronounced "Z hat"). □

REMARK.– The estimator $\hat{\beta}$ is said to be "linear", meaning that it is of the form $C\mathbf{Z}$. In our case, the matrix C is $\left(\mathbb{X}^\top \mathbb{X} \right)^{-1} \mathbb{X}^\top$. □

REMARK.– Let us return to the special case of a simple linear model:

$$Z_i = \beta_1 + \beta_2 X_i + \epsilon_i,$$

(the index "2" is omitted, simply writing X_i for X_{i2}). The empirical mean and variance of $X_1, \ldots, X_n$ are defined by $\bar{X} = \frac{1}{n} \sum_i X_i$ and $\text{var}_{emp}(X) = \frac{1}{n} \sum_i X_i^2 - \bar{X}^2$. Similarly, the empirical covariance of the X_i and Z_i is defined by $\text{covar}_{emp}(X, Z) = \frac{1}{n} \sum_i X_i Z_i - \bar{X}\bar{Z}$, where $\bar{Z} = \frac{1}{n} \sum_i Z_i$. It is easy to show that:

$$\mathbb{X}^\top \mathbb{X} = \begin{pmatrix} n & \sum_i X_i \\ \sum_i X_i & \sum_i X_i^2 \end{pmatrix}, \quad \left(\mathbb{X}^\top \mathbb{X} \right)^{-1} = \frac{1}{n^2 \text{var}_{emp}(X)} \begin{pmatrix} \sum_i X_i^2 & -\sum_i X_i \\ -\sum_i X_i & n \end{pmatrix},$$

and

$$\mathbb{X}^{\top}\mathbf{Z} = \begin{pmatrix} \sum_i Z_i \\ \sum_i X_i Z_i \end{pmatrix},$$

which gives us an expression for the least squares estimators of β_1 and β_2:

$$\hat{\beta}_2 = \frac{\text{covar}_{emp}(X, Z)}{\text{var}_{emp}(X)}, \quad \hat{\beta}_1 = \bar{Z} - \hat{\beta}_2 \bar{X}.$$

The least squares regression line is defined by:

$$\hat{Z}_i = \hat{\beta}_1 + \hat{\beta}_2 X_i = \bar{Z} + \frac{\text{covar}_{emp}(X, Z)}{\text{var}_{emp}(X)}(X_i - \bar{X}).$$

This line is plotted graphically for a set of simulated data in Figure 1.1. $\square$

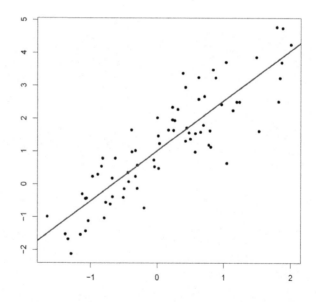

Figure 1.1. *A cloud of (simulated) points and the least squares line*

To evaluate the properties of the least squares estimator, we need to formulate additional hypotheses about the model in equation [1.1].

Accordingly, we assume that the errors ϵ_i each have mean zero and identical variance (we say that they are homoscedastic), as well as being pairwise uncorrelated. This can be summarized by the hypothesis:

$$\mathcal{H}_2 : \mathbb{E}(\mathbf{E}) = 0 \text{ and } \mathrm{var}(\mathbf{E}) = \sigma^2 I_n.$$

If the explanatory variables are themselves random variables, then these hypotheses are phrased conditionally as a function of $\mathbf{X}_i$.

If $\mathcal{H}_2$ holds, then $\hat{\beta}$ is an unbiased estimator of β. This can be shown by the following simple calculation (the explanatory variables are assumed to be fixed to simplify the notation):

$$\mathbb{E}(\hat{\beta}) = \mathbb{E}\left(\left(\mathbb{X}^\top \mathbb{X}\right)^{-1} \mathbb{X}^\top \mathbf{Z} \right) = \left(\mathbb{X}^\top \mathbb{X}\right)^{-1} \mathbb{X}^\top \mathbb{E}(\mathbf{Z})$$

$$= \left(\mathbb{X}^\top \mathbb{X}\right)^{-1} \mathbb{X}^\top \mathbb{X}\beta = \beta,$$

since $\mathbb{E}(\mathbf{Z}) = \mathbb{E}(\mathbb{X}\beta + \mathbf{E}) = \mathbb{X}\beta$ given $\mathcal{H}_2$.

We note that if $\mathcal{H}_2$ holds, then $\mathrm{var}(\mathbf{Z}) = \mathrm{var}(\mathbb{X}\beta + \mathbf{E}) = \mathrm{var}(\mathbf{E}) = \sigma^2 I_n$, which also makes the variance of $\hat{\beta}$ easy to compute:

$$\mathrm{var}(\hat{\beta}) = \mathrm{var}\left(\left(\mathbb{X}^\top \mathbb{X}\right)^{-1} \mathbb{X}^\top \mathbf{Z} \right)$$

$$= (\mathbb{X}^\top \mathbb{X})^{-1} \mathbb{X}^\top \mathrm{var}(\mathbf{Z}) \mathbb{X} (\mathbb{X}^\top \mathbb{X})^{-1}$$

$$= \sigma^2 (\mathbb{X}^\top \mathbb{X})^{-1} \mathbb{X}^\top \mathbb{X} (\mathbb{X}^\top \mathbb{X})^{-1}$$

$$= \sigma^2 (\mathbb{X}^\top \mathbb{X})^{-1}.$$

The Gauss–Markov theorem specifies the sense in which $\hat{\beta}$ is optimal:

THEOREM.– The least squares estimator has the smallest variance of any unbiased linear estimator of β.

Gauss–Markov theorem: proof

Suppose that $\tilde{\beta}$ is another unbiased linear estimator of β. We will show that $\mathrm{var}(\tilde{\beta}) \geq \mathrm{var}(\hat{\beta})$. Notationally, this matrix inequality should be interpreted as follows: $\text{var}(\tilde{\beta}) \geq \text{var}(\hat{\beta})$ whenever the matrix $\Delta := \text{var}(\tilde{\beta}) - \text{var}(\hat{\beta})$ is positive semi-definite.

The estimator $\tilde{\beta}$ is linear, so $\tilde{\beta} = A\mathbf{Z}$ for some $p \times n$ matrix A. It is also unbiased, so, for any $\beta \in \mathbb{R}^p$, we have $\mathbb{E}(\tilde{\beta}) = \mathbb{E}(A\mathbf{Z}) = A\mathbb{X}\beta = \beta$. Hence, $A\mathbb{X} = I_p$. The variance of $\tilde{\beta}$ can now be decomposed as follows:

$$\text{var}(\tilde{\beta}) = \text{var}(\tilde{\beta} - \hat{\beta} + \hat{\beta})$$

$$= \text{var}(\tilde{\beta} - \hat{\beta}) + \text{var}(\hat{\beta}) + \text{cov}(\tilde{\beta} - \hat{\beta}, \hat{\beta}) + \text{cov}(\hat{\beta}, \tilde{\beta} - \hat{\beta}).$$

We note that:

$$\text{cov}(\tilde{\beta} - \hat{\beta}, \hat{\beta}) = \text{cov}\left(A\mathbf{Z}, \left(\mathbb{X}^\top\mathbb{X}\right)^{-1}\mathbb{X}^\top\mathbf{Z}\right) - \text{var}(\hat{\beta})$$

$$= \sigma^2 A\mathbb{X}\left(\mathbb{X}^\top\mathbb{X}\right)^{-1} - \sigma^2(\mathbb{X}^\top\mathbb{X})^{-1}$$

$$= 0,$$

since $A\mathbb{X} = I_p$. It follows that $\text{var}(\tilde{\beta}) = \text{var}(\tilde{\beta} - \hat{\beta}) + \text{var}(\hat{\beta})$. Finally, given that the variance–covariance matrices are positive semi-definite, we find that $\text{var}(\tilde{\beta}) \geq \text{var}(\hat{\beta})$, as required. $\square$

REMARK.– After defining $\hat{\mathbf{Z}} := P\mathbf{Z} = \mathbb{X}\hat{\beta}$, the following expression gives an unbiased estimator of the residual variance σ^2:

$$\hat{\sigma}^2 = \frac{RSS(\hat{\beta})}{n-p} = \frac{\|\mathbf{Z} - \mathbb{X}\hat{\beta}\|^2}{n-p} = \frac{\|\mathbf{Z} - \hat{\mathbf{Z}}\|^2}{n-p}$$

(see [GUY 01] for example). The vector $\hat{\mathbf{E}} := \mathbf{Z} - \hat{\mathbf{Z}}$ is known as the residual vector. $\square$

1.3.1. *The coefficient of determination* R^2

We have seen that applying the method of least squares to the model $\mathbf{Z} = \mathbb{X}\beta + \mathbf{E}$ can be viewed as orthogonally projecting the vector $\mathbf{Z} \in \mathbb{R}^n$ onto the vector subspace $\mathcal{S}_{\mathbb{X}}$ of $\mathbb{R}^n$ spanned by the columns of the matrix $\mathbb{X}$. We define $\mathbf{1}_n$ to be the vector in $\mathbb{R}^n$ for which every component is equal to 1. The orthogonal projection of $\mathbf{Z}$ onto the line spanned by $\mathbf{1}_n$ is the vector:

$$\frac{\langle \mathbf{Z}, \mathbf{1}_n \rangle}{\langle \mathbf{1}_n, \mathbf{1}_n \rangle}\mathbf{1}_n = \bar{Z}\mathbf{1}_n.$$

This line is contained in the subspace $\mathcal{S}_{\mathbb{X}}$. By Pythagoras' theorem, the following equality holds:

$$\|\mathbf{Z} - \bar{Z}\mathbf{1}_n\|^2 = \|\mathbf{Z} - \hat{\mathbf{Z}}\|^2 + \|\hat{\mathbf{Z}} - \bar{Z}\mathbf{1}_n\|^2 = \|\hat{\mathbf{E}}\|^2 + \|\hat{\mathbf{Z}} - \bar{Z}\mathbf{1}_n\|^2,$$

which can be rewritten as:

$$\sum_{i=1}^{n}(Z_i - \bar{Z})^2 = \sum_{i=1}^{n}\hat{\epsilon}_i^2 + \sum_{i=1}^{n}(\hat{Z}_i - \bar{Z})^2,$$

where $\hat{\epsilon}_1, \ldots, \hat{\epsilon}_n$ (respectively, $\hat{Z}_1, \ldots, \hat{Z}_n$) are the components of the vector $\hat{\mathbf{E}}$ (resp. $\hat{\mathbf{Z}}$). This inequality can be interpreted as a decomposition formula for the variance of the observations: the total variance $n^{-1}\sum_{i=1}^{n}(Z_i - \bar{Z})^2$ is decomposed into the sum of the variance $n^{-1}\sum_{i=1}^{n}(\hat{Z}_i - \bar{Z})^2$ explained by the model and the residual variance $n^{-1}\sum_{i=1}^{n}\hat{\epsilon}_i^2$.

The coefficient of determination R^2 measures the goodness of fit of the model $\mathbf{Z} = \mathbb{X}\beta + \mathbf{E}$ to the data, defined as follows:

$$R^2 = \frac{\|\hat{\mathbf{Z}} - \bar{Z}\mathbf{1}_n\|^2}{\|\mathbf{Z} - \bar{Z}\mathbf{1}_n\|^2} = 1 - \frac{\|\hat{\mathbf{E}}\|^2}{\|\mathbf{Z} - \bar{Z}\mathbf{1}_n\|^2}.$$

The coefficient of determination R^2 takes values between 0 and 1. It can be interpreted as the proportion of the variability in the data that is explained by the model (if R^2 is close to 1, the model gives a good explanation of the data).

However, the coefficient of determination does not take into account the number of explanatory variables used by the model. Consequently, maximizing R^2 tends to favor models with a large number of regressors. To avoid this, the adjusted coefficient of determination is defined as follows:

$$R_a^2 = 1 - \frac{n-1}{n-p}\frac{\|\hat{\mathbf{E}}\|^2}{\|\mathbf{Z} - \bar{Z}\mathbf{1}_n\|^2} = 1 - \frac{n-1}{n-p}(1 - R^2).$$

1.4. The Gaussian linear model

To study the model in equation [1.1] in more statistical depth, for example, by constructing confidence intervals for the parameters or testing hypotheses, we need to formulate a hypothesis to specify the distribution of Z_i. We will now assume that the errors are normally distributed:

$$\mathcal{H}_3 : \mathbf{E} \sim \mathcal{N}(0, \sigma^2 I_n).$$

For each i, this means that $Z_i = \beta^\top \mathbf{X}_i + \epsilon_i$ follows the Gaussian (or normal) distribution $\mathcal{N}(\beta^\top \mathbf{X}_i, \sigma^2)$ (if the explanatory variables are themselves random variables, then Z_i given $\mathbf{X}_i$ has distribution $\mathcal{N}(\beta^\top \mathbf{X}_i, \sigma^2)$; in this case, $\mathbb{E}(Z_i|\mathbf{X}_i) = \beta^\top \mathbf{X}_i$). In vector notation:

$$\mathbf{Z} \sim \mathcal{N}(\mathbb{X}\beta, \sigma^2 I_n).$$
[1.2]

This defines the Gaussian linear model.

REMARK.– In the Gaussian case, non-correlation implies independence for observations.   □

For the Gaussian linear model, the least squares estimator of β coincides with the maximum likelihood estimator. Let us write $f_{\mathcal{N}(\beta^\top \mathbf{X}_i, \sigma^2)}$ for the density function of Y_i. Since the observations are independent, the likelihood of the pair of parameters (β, σ^2) based on the $(Z_i, \mathbf{X}_i), i = 1, \ldots, n$ is given by:

$$
\begin{aligned}
L_n(\beta, \sigma^2) &= \prod_{i=1}^{n} f_{\mathcal{N}(\beta^\top \mathbf{X}_i, \sigma^2)}(Y_i) \\
&= \prod_{i=1}^{n} \frac{1}{\sqrt{2\pi\sigma^2}} \exp\left(-\frac{1}{2\sigma^2}\left(Z_i - \beta^\top \mathbf{X}_i\right)^2\right) \\
&= \frac{1}{(2\pi\sigma^2)^{n/2}} \exp\left(-\frac{1}{2\sigma^2}\sum_{i=1}^{n}\left(Z_i - \beta^\top \mathbf{X}_i\right)^2\right) \\
&= \frac{1}{(2\pi\sigma^2)^{n/2}} \exp\left(-\frac{1}{2\sigma^2}RSS(\beta)\right).
\end{aligned}
$$
[1.3]

The maximum likelihood estimator of (β, σ^2) is defined as the pair of values $(\hat{\beta}_{mv}, \hat{\sigma}^2_{mv})$ that maximizes $L_n(\beta, \sigma^2)$. Equivalently, $(\hat{\beta}_{mv}, \hat{\sigma}^2_{mv})$ maximizes the log-likelihood $\ell_n(\beta, \sigma^2) = \ln L_n(\beta, \sigma^2)$, which is defined by:

$$\ell_n(\beta, \sigma^2) = -\frac{n}{2}\ln(2\pi\sigma^2) - \frac{1}{2\sigma^2}RSS(\beta).$$
[1.4]

By equation [1.4], given fixed σ^2, the least squares estimator $\hat{\beta}$ maximizes the likelihood and is therefore equal to $\hat{\beta}_{mv}$. We can differentiate $\partial \ell_n(\beta, \sigma^2)/\partial \sigma^2$ directly to find the maximum likelihood estimator of σ^2: $\hat{\sigma}_{mv}^2 = RSS(\hat{\beta})/n = (n - p)\hat{\sigma}^2/n$. This is a biased estimator, since

$$\mathbb{E}(\hat{\sigma}_{mv}^2) = \frac{n - p}{n}\mathbb{E}(\hat{\sigma}^2) = \frac{n - p}{n}\sigma^2,$$

but the bias tends to 0 as n tends to infinity.

The properties of $\hat{\beta}_{mv}$ and $\hat{\sigma}_{mv}^2$ (or, equivalently for the Gaussian linear model, the properties of $\hat{\beta}$ and $\hat{\sigma}^2$) are outlined in the following. But first, we give a few brief reminders about some other important distributions that can be constructed from the Gaussian distribution, as well as some results about Gaussian vectors. Readers can refer to [MON 80] for a more comprehensive presentation of these distributions.

1.4.1. *Review of some properties of Gaussian distributions*

To perform statistical inference with a Gaussian linear model, we take advantage of three other key probability distributions, together with the Gaussian distribution itself: the χ^2 distribution, Student's t-distribution and the F-distribution. The definitions of these distributions are recalled here.

1.4.1.1. *The χ^2, Student's t- and F-distributions*

DEFINITION.– Let $X_1, \ldots, X_n$ be independent identically distributed (i.i.d.) random variables with the standard Gaussian distribution (denoted $\mathcal{N}(0, 1)$). The χ^2 distribution with n degrees of freedom (denoted χ_n^2) is defined as the distribution of the sum $X_1^2 + X_2^2 + \ldots + X_n^2$.

The χ^2 distribution is itself used to define Student's t-distribution:

DEFINITION.– Let X be a random variable with distribution $\mathcal{N}(0, 1)$ and Y be a random variable with distribution χ_n^2 that is independent of X. The distribution of the variable $Z = \dfrac{X}{\sqrt{Y/n}}$ is known as Student's t-distribution with n degrees of freedom (denoted $\mathcal{T}_n$).

REMARK.– Student's t-distribution is symmetric and has mean zero. If n is sufficiently large ($n > 30$ is often recommended), then Student's t-distribution $\mathcal{T}_n$ approximates the Gaussian distribution $\mathcal{N}(0, 1)$. □

DEFINITION.– Let U_1 be a random variable with distribution $\chi^2_{n_1}$ and U_2 be a random variable independent of U_1 with distribution $\chi^2_{n_2}$. The distribution of the variable $U = \frac{U_1/n_1}{U_2/n_2}$ is known as the F-distribution with (n_1, n_2) degrees of freedom, often written F_{n_1, n_2}.

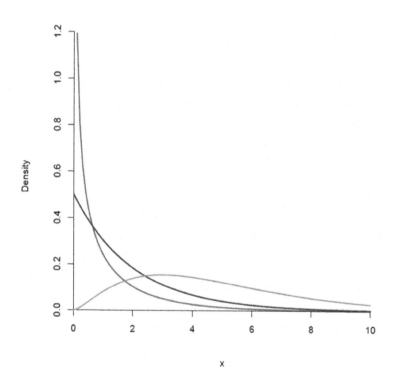

Figure 1.2. *Densities of χ^2_1 (red), χ^2_2 (blue) and χ^2_5 (gray). For a color version of the figure, please see www.iste.co.uk/dupuy/countdata.zip*

A few examples of the probability densities associated with a series of χ^2, Student's t- and F-distributions are shown in Figures 1.2, 1.3 and 1.4. The following R code [RCO 17] was used to generate Figure 1.3 and can easily be adapted to generate the two other figures.

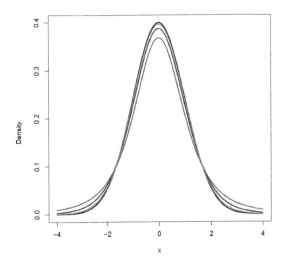

Figure 1.3. *Densities of T_3 (red), T_8 (blue), T_{30} (gray) and $\mathcal{N}(0,1)$*
(black). For a color version of the figure, please see
www.iste.co.uk/dupuy/countdata.zip

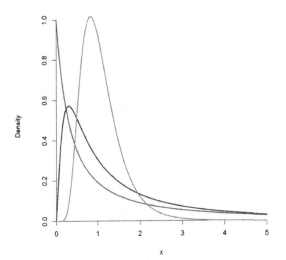

Figure 1.4. *Densities of $F_{2,1}$ (red), $F_{5,2}$ (blue) and $F_{20,25}$ (gray).*
For a color version of the figure, please see
www.iste.co.uk/dupuy/countdata.zip

```
x=seq(-4,4,length=100)
density.x=dnorm(x)   # density of the distribution N(0,1)

ddl=c(3,8,30) # number of degrees of freedom
colors=c("red","blue","darkgrey")

plot(x,density.x,type="l",lwd=2,xlab="x",ylab="Density")
for (i in 1:3){
   lines(x,dt(x,ddl[i]),lwd=2,col=colors[i])
}
```

1.4.1.2. *Review of Gaussian vectors*

A random vector X taking values in $\mathbb{R}^p$ with mean $\mathbb{E}(X) = m \in \mathbb{R}^p$ and variance–covariance matrix $\Sigma = \mathbb{E}[(X - m)(X - m)^\top]$ is said to follow a multivariate Gaussian distribution (or is said to be a Gaussian vector) if it has the probability density function

$$f(x) = \frac{1}{(2\pi)^{p/2}\sqrt{\det(\Sigma)}} \exp\left(-\frac{1}{2}(x - m)^\top \Sigma^{-1}(x - m)\right),$$

where $x = (x_1, \ldots, x_p) \in \mathbb{R}^p$ (the matrix Σ has size $p \times p$ and is assumed to be invertible). Notationally, we write that $X \sim \mathcal{N}(m, \Sigma)$.

Gaussian vectors have the following key property: if $X \sim \mathcal{N}(m, \Sigma)$ is a Gaussian vector in $\mathbb{R}^p$ and $A : \mathbb{R}^p \to \mathbb{R}^q$ is a linear mapping, then $AX \sim \mathcal{N}(Am, A\Sigma A^\top)$ in $\mathbb{R}^q$. If $X \sim \mathcal{N}(m, \Sigma)$ is a Gaussian vector in $\mathbb{R}^p$ and Σ is invertible, then $(X - m)^\top \Sigma^{-1}(X - m) \sim \chi_p^2$.

Cochran's theorem is recalled below without proof. This theorem guarantees that any decomposition of a Gaussian vector in $\mathbb{R}^p$ onto orthogonal subspaces yields independent random variables. Furthermore, we can give the distribution of each random variable.

THEOREM.– Let Y be a Gaussian vector with distribution $\mathcal{N}(m, \sigma^2 I_p)$, $\mathcal{S}$ be a q-dimensional subspace of $\mathbb{R}^p$, P be the matrix of orthogonal projection onto $\mathcal{S}$ and $P_\perp = I_p - P$ be the matrix of orthogonal projection onto $\mathcal{S}^\perp$, the orthogonal complement of $\mathcal{S}$ in $\mathbb{R}^p$. Then:

1) $PY \sim \mathcal{N}(Pm, \sigma^2 P)$ and $P_\perp Y \sim \mathcal{N}(P_\perp m, \sigma^2 P_\perp)$,

2) the vectors PY and $P_\perp Y = Y - PY$ are independent,

3) $\frac{\|P(Y-m)\|^2}{\sigma^2} \sim \chi_q^2$ and $\frac{\|P_\perp(Y-m)\|^2}{\sigma^2} \sim \chi_{p-q}^2$.

Let us now return to discussing the properties of the maximum likelihood estimators in the Gaussian linear model.

1.4.2. *Distributions of estimators*

THEOREM.– *The estimators* $\hat{\beta}$ *and* $\hat{\sigma}^2$ *in the Gaussian linear model* [1.2] *satisfy the following properties:*

1) $\hat{\beta} \sim \mathcal{N}(\beta, \sigma^2(\mathbb{X}^\top \mathbb{X})^{-1})$,

2) $(n-p)\hat{\sigma}^2/\sigma^2 \sim \chi_{n-p}^2$,

3) $\hat{\beta}$ and $\hat{\sigma}^2$ are independent.

PROOF.– To show Property 1, we observe that $\hat{\beta}$ is the image of the Gaussian vector $\mathbf{Z}$ under a linear mapping. Hence, it is itself a Gaussian vector with the mean and variance stated previously.

For Property 2, we recall that $\mathcal{S}_{\mathbb{X}}$ denotes the p-dimensional subspace of $\mathbb{R}^n$ spanned by the column vectors of the matrix $\mathbb{X}$. We also recall that P is the matrix of orthogonal projection onto $\mathcal{S}_{\mathbb{X}}$ and write $P_\perp$ for the matrix of orthogonal projection onto the orthogonal complement of $\mathcal{S}_{\mathbb{X}}$ (which is an $(n-p)$-dimensional subspace of $\mathbb{R}^n$). Then:

$$\hat{\mathbf{E}} = \mathbf{Z} - P\mathbf{Z} = P_\perp \mathbf{Z} = P_\perp \mathbf{E},$$

since $\mathbf{Z} = \mathbb{X}\beta + \mathbf{E}$ and $\mathbb{X}\beta \in \mathcal{S}_{\mathbb{X}}$. By Cochran's theorem, it follows that

$$\frac{(n-p)}{\sigma^2}\hat{\sigma}^2 = \frac{\|\mathbf{Z} - P\mathbf{Z}\|^2}{\sigma^2} = \frac{\|\hat{\mathbf{E}}\|^2}{\sigma^2}$$

$$= \frac{\|P_\perp \mathbf{E}\|^2}{\sigma^2} = \frac{\|P_\perp(\mathbf{E} - \mathbb{E}(\mathbf{E}))\|^2}{\sigma^2} \sim \chi_{n-p}^2.$$

Finally, for Property 3, we note that $\hat{\beta}$ is a random vector that can be written as a function of $P\mathbf{Z}$:

$$\hat{\beta} = (\mathbb{X}^\top \mathbb{X})^{-1} \mathbb{X}^\top \mathbf{Z}$$
$$= (\mathbb{X}^\top \mathbb{X})^{-1} \mathbb{X}^\top \underbrace{(\mathbb{X}(\mathbb{X}^\top \mathbb{X})^{-1} \mathbb{X}^\top)}_{P} \mathbf{Z}$$
$$= (\mathbb{X}^\top \mathbb{X})^{-1} \mathbb{X}^\top P\mathbf{Z}.$$

Similarly, $\hat{\sigma}^2 = \frac{\|\mathbf{Z} - P\mathbf{Z}\|^2}{n-p}$ is a random variable that can be expressed as a function of $\mathbf{Z} - P\mathbf{Z}$. By Cochran's theorem, $P\mathbf{Z}$ and $\mathbf{Z} - P\mathbf{Z}$ are independent. Functions of independent variables are independent, so $\hat{\beta}$ and $\hat{\sigma}^2$ are independent, as required. $\square$

REMARK.– The estimator $\hat{\beta}$ in the Gaussian linear model minimizes the variance over the set of (possibly nonlinear) unbiased estimators of β. $\square$

Properties 1, 2 and 3 are valuable tools when we want to construct confidence intervals/regions for the model parameters or test statistics for these parameters. For example, the following result allows us to construct confidence intervals and test statistics for the coefficient β_i ($i = 1, \ldots, p$).

We define $[(\mathbb{X}^\top \mathbb{X})^{-1}]_{i,i}$ as the i-th term on the diagonal of the matrix $(\mathbb{X}^\top \mathbb{X})^{-1}$. Then, for all $i = 1, \ldots, p$:

$$T_i = \frac{\hat{\beta}_i - \beta_i}{\hat{\sigma}\sqrt{[(\mathbb{X}^\top \mathbb{X})^{-1}]_{i,i}}} \sim \mathcal{T}_{n-p}. \qquad [1.5]$$

This result is easy to show. By Property 1, $\frac{\hat{\beta}_i - \beta_i}{\sigma\sqrt{[(\mathbb{X}^\top \mathbb{X})^{-1}]_{i,i}}} \sim \mathcal{N}(0, 1)$. By Property 3, $\hat{\beta}_i$ and $\hat{\sigma}^2$ are independent. Therefore, by Property 2, the variable:

$$\frac{\dfrac{\hat{\beta}_i - \beta_i}{\sigma\sqrt{[(\mathbb{X}^\top \mathbb{X})^{-1}]_{i,i}}}}{\sqrt{(n-p)\dfrac{\hat{\sigma}^2}{\sigma^2}/(n-p)}} = \frac{\hat{\beta}_i - \beta_i}{\hat{\sigma}\sqrt{[(\mathbb{X}^\top \mathbb{X})^{-1}]_{i,i}}}$$

has distribution $\mathcal{T}_{n-p}$.

1.4.3. *Confidence intervals*

This section gives examples of confidence intervals: for a regression coefficient β_i, for the variance σ^2 and for a prediction. This topic is discussed in more depth by [AZA 06, COR 07].

1.4.3.1. *Confidence interval for a regression coefficient*

Let $\alpha \in]0, 1[$, and we write $t_{n-p}(u)$ for the quantile of order u of the distribution $\mathcal{T}_{n-p}$, defined by $\mathbb{P}(\mathcal{T}_{n-p} \leq t_{n-p}(u)) = u$. From equation [1.5], we can construct the $(1 - \alpha)$ bilateral confidence interval for β_i $(i = 1, \ldots, p)$ as follows:

$$\Bigg[\hat{\beta}_i - t_{n-p}(1 - \alpha/2)\hat{\sigma}\sqrt{[(\mathbb{X}^\top\mathbb{X})^{-1}]_{i,i}};$$

$$\hat{\beta}_i + t_{n-p}(1 - \alpha/2)\hat{\sigma}\sqrt{[(\mathbb{X}^\top\mathbb{X})^{-1}]_{i,i}} \Bigg].$$

REMARK.– Considered separately, the confidence intervals of the β_i do not account for any dependence between the $\hat{\beta}_i$. This dependence can be incorporated by constructing confidence regions for multiple parameters simultaneously, which is more precise than simply juxtaposing multiple individual confidence intervals. More details can be found in [COR 07].   □

1.4.3.2. *Confidence interval for the variance σ^2*

Let $c_{n-p}(u)$ be the quantile of u of the distribution χ^2_{n-p}, defined by $\mathbb{P}(\chi^2_{n-p} \leq c_{n-p}(u)) = u$. The $(1 - \alpha)$ bilateral confidence interval for σ^2 can be defined as follows:

$$\left[\frac{(n - p)\hat{\sigma}^2}{c_{n-p}(1 - \alpha/2)} ; \frac{(n - p)\hat{\sigma}^2}{c_{n-p}(\alpha/2)} \right].$$

1.4.3.3. *Prediction interval*

Suppose that the model $\mathbf{Z} \sim \mathcal{N}(\mathbb{X}\beta, \sigma^2 I_n)$, where $\beta \in \mathbb{R}^p$, was estimated from n observations $(Z_1, \mathbf{X}_1), \ldots, (Z_n, \mathbf{X}_n)$. We consider another individual (with index $n + 1$) and write $\mathbf{X}_{n+1} = (1, X_{n+1,2}, \ldots, X_{n+1,p})^\top$ for its vector of covariables. Suppose that we wish to predict the response Z_{n+1} of the model $Z_{n+1} = \beta^\top \mathbf{X}_{n+1} + \epsilon_{n+1}$, where $\epsilon_{n+1} \sim \mathcal{N}(0, \sigma^2)$ at this individual. We shall assume that Z_{n+1} is independent of $Z_1, \ldots, Z_n$.

A natural approach to predict Z_{n+1} is to define:

$$\hat{Z}^p_{n+1} = \hat{\beta}^\top \mathbf{X}_{n+1},$$

where $\hat{\beta}$ is the maximum likelihood estimator of β obtained from the n observations $(Z_i, \mathbf{X}_i), i = 1, \ldots, n$. The prediction error

$$Z_{n+1} - \hat{Z}^p_{n+1} = (\beta - \hat{\beta})^\top \mathbf{X}_{n+1} + \epsilon_{n+1}$$

follows a Gaussian distribution with mean

$$\mathbb{E}(Z_{n+1} - \hat{Z}^p_{n+1}) = 0$$

and variance

$$\mathrm{var}(Z_{n+1} - \hat{Z}^p_{n+1}) = \mathrm{var}\left((\beta - \hat{\beta})^\top \mathbf{X}_{n+1} + \epsilon_{n+1}\right)$$
$$= \mathbf{X}^\top_{n+1}\mathrm{var}(\beta - \hat{\beta})\mathbf{X}_{n+1} + \sigma^2$$
$$= \sigma^2\left[\mathbf{X}^\top_{n+1}(\mathbb{X}^\top\mathbb{X})^{-1}\mathbf{X}_{n+1} + 1\right].$$

Therefore:

$$N := \frac{Z_{n+1} - \hat{Z}^p_{n+1}}{\sigma\sqrt{\mathbf{X}^\top_{n+1}(\mathbb{X}^\top\mathbb{X})^{-1}\mathbf{X}_{n+1} + 1}} \sim \mathcal{N}(0, 1).$$

The quantities $\hat{\sigma}^2$ and $(Z_{n+1} - \hat{Z}^p_{n+1})$ are independent, since $\hat{\sigma}^2$ only depends on the $Z_1, \ldots, Z_n$ and so is independent of ϵ_{n+1}, and $\hat{\sigma}^2$ is also independent of $\hat{\beta}$. Furthermore, $D := (n - p)\hat{\sigma}^2/\sigma^2 \sim \chi^2_{n-p}$. Hence, by construction, the variable

$$\frac{N}{\sqrt{\frac{D}{n-p}}} = \frac{Z_{n+1} - \hat{Z}^p_{n+1}}{\hat{\sigma}\sqrt{\mathbf{X}^\top_{n+1}(\mathbb{X}^\top\mathbb{X})^{-1}\mathbf{X}_{n+1} + 1}}$$

follows Student's t-distribution $\mathcal{T}_{n-p}$. From this, we can deduce a $(1 - \alpha)$ prediction interval for Z_{n+1}:

$$\left[\hat{Z}^p_{n+1} - t_{n-p}(1 - \alpha/2)\hat{\sigma}\sqrt{\mathbf{X}^\top_{n+1}(\mathbb{X}^\top\mathbb{X})^{-1}\mathbf{X}_{n+1} + 1} \; ; \right.$$

$$\left. \hat{Z}^p_{n+1} + t_{n-p}(1 - \alpha/2)\hat{\sigma}\sqrt{\mathbf{X}^\top_{n+1}(\mathbb{X}^\top\mathbb{X})^{-1}\mathbf{X}_{n+1} + 1} \right].$$

1.4.4. Hypothesis tests

This section states a few classical tests for the Gaussian linear model (nullity test for a single regression coefficient, test between nested models). More details can be found in [AZA 06, COR 07].

1.4.4.1. Test for a single component of β (Student's t-test)

Let b be a known real number. Suppose that we wish to test $H_0 : \beta_i = b$ against $H_1 : \beta_i \neq b$ (the most frequently encountered situation is the case where $b = 0$, which allows us to test the non-significance of an explanatory variable). By equation [1.5], under H_0, the variable

$$T_i = \frac{\hat{\beta}_i - b}{\hat{\sigma}\sqrt{[(\mathbb{X}^\top\mathbb{X})^{-1}]_{i,i}}}$$

has the distribution $\mathcal{T}_{n-p}$. The region of rejection of H_0 for a significance level of α can be defined as:

$$\mathcal{R}_\alpha = \{|T_i| \geq t_{n-p}(1 - \alpha/2)\}.$$

1.4.4.2. Test between nested models (F-test)

Suppose that we want to test whether q parameters β_i are simultaneously null in the model:

$$\mathbf{Z} = \mathbb{X}\beta + \mathbf{E}, \quad \mathbf{E} \sim \mathcal{N}(0, \sigma^2 I_n), \quad \beta \in \mathbb{R}^p. \quad\quad [1.6]$$

For example, we might want to test the significance of a categorical variable with three or more values, which can be rephrased in terms of several indicator variables.

To simplify the notation, assume without loss of generality that we are testing the nullity of the q last coefficients of β. The test problem can be stated as $H_0 : \beta_{p-q+1} = \ldots = \beta_p = 0$ against H_1 : there exists $i \in \{p-q+1, \ldots, p\}$ such that $\beta_i \neq 0$.

Under H_0, the model becomes:

$$\mathbf{Z} = \mathbb{X}^* \beta^* + \mathbf{E}^*, \quad \mathbf{E}^* \sim \mathcal{N}(0, \sigma^2 I_n), \tag{1.7}$$

where $\mathbb{X}^*$ is an $n \times (p-q)$ matrix containing the $(p-q)$ first columns of $\mathbb{X}$ and β^* is a vector of size $(p-q)$ containing the regression coefficients. The $(p-q)$ columns of $\mathbb{X}^*$ generate a $(p-q)$-dimensional vector subspace $\mathcal{S}_{\mathbb{X}^*}$ of $\mathbb{R}^n$. This subspace is contained in $\mathcal{S}_{\mathbb{X}}$ (the vector subspace spanned by the columns of $\mathbb{X}$).

We recall that estimating β in the model from equation [1.6] (respectively β^* in the model from equation [1.7]) by the method of least squares is essentially equivalent to projecting $\mathbf{Z}$ onto $\mathcal{S}_{\mathbb{X}}$ to find $\hat{\mathbf{Z}} := \mathbb{X}\hat{\beta}$ (respectively onto $\mathcal{S}_{\mathbb{X}^*}$ to find $\hat{\mathbf{Z}}^* = \mathbb{X}^*\hat{\beta}^*$).

The F-test is inspired by the following intuition: if the projections $\hat{\mathbf{Z}}$ and $\hat{\mathbf{Z}}^*$ are "close" (i.e. if the norm $\|\hat{\mathbf{Z}} - \hat{\mathbf{Z}}^*\|^2$ is small), then the model from equation [1.7] performs "almost as well as" the more comprehensive model from equation [1.6], while requiring fewer explanatory variables. The model from equation [1.7] is therefore preferable, since it is simpler. This leads us to define the test statistic:

$$F = \frac{\|\hat{\mathbf{Z}} - \hat{\mathbf{Z}}^*\|^2/q}{\|\mathbf{Z} - \hat{\mathbf{Z}}\|^2/(n-p)}.$$

REMARK.– The division of $\|\hat{\mathbf{Z}} - \hat{\mathbf{Z}}^*\|^2$ by $\|\mathbf{Z} - \hat{\mathbf{Z}}\|^2$ can be interpreted as a normalization operation that eliminates the measurement units when computing $\|\hat{\mathbf{Z}} - \hat{\mathbf{Z}}^*\|^2$. Similarly, each of the terms $\|\hat{\mathbf{Z}} - \hat{\mathbf{Z}}^*\|^2$ and $\|\mathbf{Z} - \hat{\mathbf{Z}}\|^2$ is normalized by its number of degrees of freedom. □

Given H_0, the F-statistic follows the F-distribution $F_{q,n-p}$. From this, we can deduce a region of rejection for H_0 (also known as the critical region) for a significance level of α:

$$\mathcal{R}_\alpha = \{F \geq f_{q,n-p}(1 - \alpha)\},$$

where $f_{q,n-p}(1 - \alpha)$ denotes the quantile of order $(1 - \alpha)$ of the distribution $F_{q,n-p}$, defined by $\mathbb{P}(F_{q,n-p} \leq f_{q,n-p}(1 - \alpha)) = 1 - \alpha$.

REMARK.– Intuitively, it is not surprising that $F \sim F_{q,n-p}$ under H_0, since F is the ratio of the squares of two norms. By Cochran's theorem, it can be shown that the numerator and denominator of F both follow χ^2 distributions and are mutually independent (see, for example, [COR 07]). □

REMARK.– The F-test is identical to the maximum likelihood-ratio test. The statistic of the latter is defined in general as $\sup_{H_0} L_n(\beta, \sigma^2)/\sup_{H_1} L_n(\beta, \sigma^2)$, where L_n is the likelihood [1.3]. □

There are two special cases of the F-test that need to be discussed separately: the F-test of overall significance and the nullity test for a single coefficient β_i.

F-test of overall significance. Suppose that we want to test the nullity of every coefficient of the model from equation [1.6], except the constant. The test problem can be stated as $H_0 : \beta_2 = \ldots = \beta_p = 0$ against H_1 : there exists $i \in \{2, \ldots, p\}$ such that $\beta_i \neq 0$. Here, q is equal to $p - 1$ and $\mathcal{S}_{\mathbb{X}^*}$ is spanned by the vector $\mathbf{1}_n \in \mathbb{R}^n$. The orthogonal projection of $\mathbf{Z}$ onto $\mathcal{S}_{\mathbb{X}^*}$ is the vector $\hat{\mathbf{Z}}^* = \bar{Z}\mathbf{1}_n$. The F-statistic is:

$$F = \frac{\|\hat{\mathbf{Z}} - \bar{Z}\mathbf{1}_n\|^2/(p-1)}{\|\mathbf{Z} - \hat{\mathbf{Z}}\|^2/(n-p)}.$$

Given H_0, F follows the F-distribution $F_{p-1,n-p}$. From this, we deduce a region of rejection of H_0 at the level α:

$$\mathcal{R}_\alpha = \{F \geq f_{p-1,n-p}(1 - \alpha)\}.$$

We note that F can also be expressed in terms of the coefficient of determination R^2: $F = \frac{R^2}{1-R^2}\frac{n-p}{p-1}$. For this reason, this test is sometimes called the R^2 test.

Nullity test for a single coefficient. Suppose now that we only want to test the nullity of a single coefficient β_i. The test problem can be stated as H_0 : $\beta_i = 0$ against $H_1 : \beta_i \neq 0$. This is the bilateral significance test of the i-th covariable. Here, q is equal to 1 and F follows the F-distribution $F_{1,n-p}$ under H_0. We deduce the region of rejection of H_0 at the level α:

$$\mathcal{R}_\alpha = \{F \geq f_{1,n-p}(1-\alpha)\}.$$

This test can be shown to be equivalent to Student's t-test and has the critical region $\mathcal{R}_\alpha = \{|T_i| \geq t_{n-p}(1-\alpha/2)\}$ described previously.

1.5. Linear models in R

In the statistical programming environment R, we can use the function `lm` to perform model fitting. We will illustrate the use of this function on a data set provided by the AER package that accompanies the book [KLE 08]. Before doing anything else, we need to load this package in R by running the command:

```
library(AER)
```

The data from this package were collected by a study performed in 1988 by the US Census Bureau on 28,155 male workers between 18 and 70 years of age. For each individual, a series of variables were recorded, including:

– weekly salary (in US dollars): `wage`,

– duration of education (in years): `education`,

– (estimated) duration of professional experience (in years): `experience`,

– a variable indicating whether the individual was working part-time at the time of the study: `parttime` (taking values yes/no).

The R command:

```
help(CPS1988)
```

opens up an online documentation page that gives a full description of the data. For a summary overview, we can instead run:

```
data(CPS1988)
str(CPS1988)
```

which returns the output:

```
'data.frame':    28155 obs. of   7 variables:
 $ wage      : num   355 123 370 755 594 ...
 $ education : int   7 12 9 11 12 16 8 12 12 14 ...
 $ experience: int   45 1 9 46 36 22 51 34 0 18 ...
 $ ethnicity:Factor w/2levels"cauc","afam":1 1 1 1 1 ...
 $ smsa : Factor w/2 levels "no","yes": 2 2 2 2 2 2 2 ...
 $ region    : Factor w/ 4 levels "northeast","midwest"
     ,..: 1 1 1 1 1 1 1 1 1 1 ...
 $ parttime:Factor w/2levels"no","yes":1 2 1 1 1 1 1...
```

The dataset contains 28,155 observations and 7 variables: the quantitative variable wage, the integer variables education and experience, and the qualitative variables (or factors) ethnicity, smsa (for "Standard Metropolitan Statistical Area"), region, and parttime. There is also some information about the levels of each factor: numbers and names. The first few observations from the dataset can be displayed as follows:

```
head(CPS1988)
```

which returns:

```
  wage education experience ethnicity smsa   region parttime
1 354.94       7         45      cauc  yes northeast       no
2 123.46      12          1      cauc  yes northeast      yes
3 370.37       9          9      cauc  yes northeast       no
4 754.94      11         46      cauc  yes northeast       no
5 593.54      12         36      cauc  yes northeast       no
6 377.23      16         22      cauc  yes northeast       no
```

A brief descriptive analysis of the data can be displayed by running the following command:

```
summary(CPS1988)
```

which returns:

```
        wage                  education          experience  ethnicity
 Min.    :    50.05   Min.   : 0.00   Min.   :-4.0   cauc:25923
 1st Qu.:   308.64   1st Qu.:12.00   1st Qu.: 8.0   afam: 2232
 Median :   522.32   Median :12.00   Median :16.0
 Mean    :   603.73   Mean   :13.07   Mean   :18.2
 3rd Qu.:   783.48   3rd Qu.:15.00   3rd Qu.:27.0
 Max.    :18777.20   Max.   :18.00   Max.   :63.0

 smsa             region          parttime
 no : 7223   northeast:6441   no :25631
 yes:20932   midwest  :6863   yes: 2524
             south    :8760
             west     :6091
```

The code:

```
par(mfrow = c(1,2))
hist(wage,freq=F,col="darkgrey")
hist(log(wage),freq=F,col="darkgrey")
lines(density(log(wage)),col="blue",lwd=2)
```

generates histograms of wage and log(wage) and overlays the latter with an estimate of the probability density of log(wage) obtained by the method of kernel density estimation.

Suppose that we want to construct a linear regression model of the salary with respect to the explanatory variables education, experience, and parttime. It makes sense to do this by modeling log(wage), since it is less asymmetric than the original variable wage. Our model can be stated as follows:

$$\log(\texttt{wage}) = \beta_1 + \beta_2 \texttt{education} + \beta_3 \texttt{experience} + \beta_4 \texttt{parttime} + \epsilon.$$

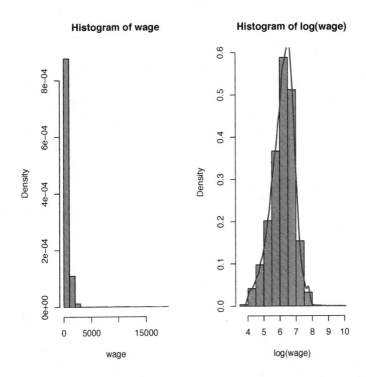

Figure 1.5. *Histograms of wage (left) and log(wage) (right)*

In R, we can fit this model to the data using the lm function:

```
cps_lm=lm(log(wage)~education+experience+parttime,data=
    CPS1988)
```

To display the results, execute the command:

```
summary(cps_lm)
```

which returns[1]:

---

1 We do not attempt to interpret this output here. The purpose of this section is simply to present a few useful R functions for fitting linear models.

```
Call:
lm(formula=log(wage)~education+experience+parttime,data=
    CPS1988)

Residuals:
    Min      1Q  Median      3Q     Max
-2.6655 -0.3245  0.0396  0.3572  4.0359

Coefficients:
              Estimate Std. Error t value Pr(>|t|)
(Intercept)  4.6847138  0.0180518  259.51  <2e-16 ***
education    0.0971624  0.0011959   81.25  <2e-16 ***
experience   0.0171689  0.0002663   64.47  <2e-16 ***
parttimeyes -1.0739747  0.0116808  -91.94  <2e-16 ***
---
Signif.codes: 0'***' 0.001 '**' 0.01'*' 0.05 '.' 0.1 '' 1

Residual standard error: 0.557 on 28151 degrees of
    freedom
Multiple R-squared:  0.3946,    Adjusted R-squared:
    0.3946
F-statistic:   6117 on 3 and 28151 DF,  p-value: < 2.2e-16
```

The "Estimate" column lists the estimates of $\beta_1, \ldots, \beta_4$. The "Residual standard error" gives the value of $\hat{\sigma}$ (estimated σ from $\epsilon \sim \mathcal{N}(0, \sigma^2)$). The "Std. error" column (short for "standard error") shows the estimated standard deviations of the estimators of each β_i. The result of Student's t-test for the nullity of β_i is shown in the "t value" column. The t-statistic is defined as the ratio "Estimate / Std. error" and follows a distribution of the form $\mathcal{T}_{n-p}$ given the null hypothesis (with $n = 28,155$ and $p = 4$ in this example). Thus, for a test with a significance level of α, the absolute values of the numbers in the "t value" column can be compared with the quantile of order $1 - \alpha/2$ of the distribution $\mathcal{T}_{28151}$ (or the Gaussian distribution $\mathcal{N}(0,1)$) (in practice, we often choose $\alpha = 0.05$). In our case, R lists the "p-value" (described as "Pr(> |t|)"), which is defined as the probability that the distribution of the test statistic given H_0 yields a value higher than the observed test statistic. We reject H_0 whenever the p-value is lower than the significance level α of the test. Finally, the output gives the values of the coefficient of determination and the adjusted coefficient of determination, as well as the F-test of overall significance for $H_0 : \beta_2 = \beta_3 = \beta_4 = 0$.

Suppose now that we wish to test the null hypothesis $H_0 : \beta_3 = \beta_4 = 0$ against the alternative hypothesis $H_1 : \beta_3 \neq 0$ or $\beta_4 \neq 0$. In other words, we are comparing the nested models:

$$\log(\texttt{wage}) = \beta_1 + \beta_2 \texttt{education} + \beta_3 \texttt{experience} + \beta_4 \texttt{parttime} + \epsilon,$$

and:

$$\log(\texttt{wage}) = \beta_1 + \beta_2 \texttt{education} + \epsilon.$$

In R, the F-test is implemented by the anova function:

```
cps=lm(log(wage)~education,data=CPS1988)
anova(cps,cps_lm)
```

which returns:

```
Analysis of Variance Table

Model 1: log(wage) ~ education
Model 2: log(wage) ~ education + experience + parttime
  Res.Df      RSS Df Sum of Sq      F    Pr(>F)
1  28153  13063.3
2  28151   8734.6  2    4328.7 6975.6 < 2.2e-16 ***
---
Signif.codes: 0'***' 0.001 '**' 0.01'*' 0.05 '.' 0.1 '' 1
```

Again, R gives the value of the test statistic ("F" column) and the corresponding p-value ("Pr(>F)" column).

REMARK.– This test can alternatively be applied in R by running the update function, which takes the object cps_lm as an argument and applies the changes indicated by the user to the corresponding model. The syntax of this command is as follows:

```
cps=update(cps_lm,formula=.~.-experience-parttime)
anova(cps,cps_lm)
```

The waldtest function from the lmtest package [ZEI 02] provides an even more concise way of implementing this test. The command:

```
waldtest(cps_lm,formula=.~. -experience-parttime,test="F"
    )
```

returns the output:

```
Wald test

Model 1: log(wage) ~ education + experience + parttime
Model 2: log(wage) ~ education
  Res.Df Df       F      Pr(>F)
1  28151
2  28153 -2 6975.6 < 2.2e-16 ***
---
Signif. codes: 0 '***' 0.001 '**' 0.01 '*' 0.05 '.' 0.1 '
    ' 1
```

□

The confint function computes confidence intervals for the parameters. For example, the command:

```
confint(cps_lm,level=0.95)
```

returns 0.95 confidence intervals for the β_i:

```
                  2.5 %        97.5 %
(Intercept)  4.64933142   4.72009617
education    0.09481839   0.09950642
experience   0.01664690   0.01769084
parttimeyes -1.09686968  -1.05107967
```

Suppose that we need a confidence interval to predict log(wage) for an individual with education=10, experience=15 and parttime="no". The command:

```
predict(cps_lm,newdata=data.frame(education=10,experience
    =15, parttime="no"),interval="prediction",level=0.95)
```

returns a prediction (fit), as well as the lower (lwr) and upper (upr) bounds of a 0.95 confidence interval:

```
           fit       lwr       upr
1  5.913871  4.822026  7.005716
```

1.6. Asymptotic properties

In this section, we briefly state a few asymptotic properties of $\hat{\beta}$ and $\hat{\sigma}^2$ (i.e. properties that are satisfied when the sample size n tends to infinity). A more detailed discussion of the asymptotics of the linear model is given in [ANT 92, AZA 06, GUY 01].

We consider the model:

$$Z_i = \beta^\top \mathbf{X}_i + \epsilon_i, \quad i = 1, \ldots, n,$$

and suppose that the ϵ_i are i.i.d. with mean zero and variance σ^2. We do not assume that the ϵ_i follow any specific distribution. In particular, we do not assume that they are normally distributed.

REMARK.– The design matrix depends on n: it has size $n \times p$ (where $p < n$). We did not need to explicitly highlight this dependence in the notation earlier, since it was not relevant. However, we shall now keep track of it by writing $\mathbf{Z} = \mathbb{X}_n \beta + \mathbf{E}$. □

Our first theorem requires the hypotheses $\mathcal{H}_1 : \mathbb{X}_n$ has full rank p; and $\mathcal{H}_2 : \mathbb{E}(\mathbf{E}) = 0$ and var$(\mathbf{E}) = \sigma^2 I_n$.

THEOREM.– If the hypotheses $\mathcal{H}_1$ and $\mathcal{H}_2$ are satisfied and $\left(\mathbb{X}_n^\top \mathbb{X}_n\right)^{-1}$ tends to 0 as n tends to infinity, then $\hat{\beta} = \left(\mathbb{X}_n^\top \mathbb{X}_n\right)^{-1} \mathbb{X}_n^\top \mathbf{Z}$ converges in probability to β (we say that $\hat{\beta}$ is a weakly consistent estimator of β, or just a consistent estimator).

PROOF.– The estimator $\hat{\beta}$ is unbiased and var$(\hat{\beta}) = \sigma^2 (\mathbb{X}_n^\top \mathbb{X}_n)^{-1}$. If $\left(\mathbb{X}_n^\top \mathbb{X}_n\right)^{-1}$ tends to 0, then var$(\hat{\beta})$ tends to 0 and $\hat{\beta}$ tends to β in quadratic mean and hence in probability. □

The next question is of course whether $\hat{\beta}$ converges in distribution. It can be shown that the asymptotic distribution of $\hat{\beta}$ is Gaussian, which allows us to construct asymptotic confidence intervals and asymptotic tests for β without assuming that the observations are normally distributed.

We recall that the matrix of orthogonal projection onto the vector subspace spanned by the columns of $\mathbb{X}_n$ can be expressed as $H_n = \mathbb{X}_n \left(\mathbb{X}_n^\top \mathbb{X}_n\right)^{-1} \mathbb{X}_n^\top$, and write $\|H_n\| = \max_{i=1,\ldots,n} |H_{n,ii}|$, where $H_{n,ii}$ is the i-the term on the diagonal of the matrix H_n.

Proofs of the following two theorems can, for example, be found in [AZA 06].

THEOREM.– *Suppose that the hypotheses* $\mathcal{H}_1$ *and* $\mathcal{H}_2$ *are satisfied, the* ϵ_i *are i.i.d.,* $\frac{1}{n}(\mathbb{X}_n^\top \mathbb{X}_n)$ *tends to a positive-definite matrix* Q *and* $\|H_n\|$ *tends to 0 as* n *tends to infinity. Then,* $\sqrt{n}(\hat{\beta} - \beta)$ *converges in distribution to the Gaussian vector* $\mathcal{N}(0, \sigma^2 Q^{-1})$.

We need a convergent estimator of σ^2 in order to construct asymptotic confidence intervals and tests for β.

THEOREM.– *Suppose that* $\mathcal{H}_1$ *and* $\mathcal{H}_2$ *are satisfied and that the* ϵ_i *are i.i.d. Then,* $\hat{\sigma}^2$ *converges in probability to* σ^2.

There are many other aspects of the linear model that deserve to be studied in their own right: model validation, variable selection techniques, generalized least squares when var($\mathbf{E}$) is an arbitrary symmetric positive-definite matrix, regression on qualitative variables and so on. Readers interested in these topics are welcome to find out more in the very comprehensive presentations given by [AZA 06, COR 07, GUY 01].

Linear models perform especially well in the case of a quantitative real response variable. However, they tend to struggle to explain discrete variables (binomial, multinomial, Poisson, etc.). Generalized linear models are more suitable for these cases; we shall study them in the next chapter.

Generalized Linear Models

The first concept introduced in this chapter is that of exponential families, which play a key role in the definition of generalized linear models.

2.1. Exponential families

2.1.1. *Definition, mean and variance*

We recall that a parametric statistical model is defined as a family of probability distributions indexed by many finite parameters. A parametric statistical model $(P_{\theta,\phi})_{\theta,\phi}$ is said to be an exponential model if $P_{\theta,\phi}$ has a probability density function (with respect to some dominating measure: the Lebesgue measure on $\mathbb{R}$ or the counting measure on $\mathbb{N}$) of the form:

$$f(y;\theta,\phi) = \exp\left(\frac{\theta y - b(\theta)}{a(\phi)} + c(y,\phi)\right), \qquad [2.1]$$

where $a(\cdot)$, $b(\cdot)$ and $c(\cdot,\cdot)$ are functions determined by the model (binomial, Poisson, etc.). The family of density functions $(f(y;\theta,\phi))_{\theta,\phi}$ is said to be an exponential family.

REMARK.– In equation [2.1], the parameter θ is known as the canonical parameter. □

Let Y be a random variable with the density function in equation [2.1], and we define $\dot{b}(\theta) = \frac{\partial}{\partial\theta}b(\theta)$ and $\ddot{b}(\theta) = \frac{\partial^2}{\partial\theta^2}b(\theta)$. Then:

$$\mathbb{E}(Y) = \dot{b}(\theta) \quad \text{and} \quad \text{var}(Y) = \ddot{b}(\theta)a(\phi). \qquad [2.2]$$

REMARK.– If we write $\mu := \mathbb{E}(Y) = \dot{b}(\theta)$, then $\ddot{b}(\theta) = \frac{\partial \dot{b}(\theta)}{\partial \theta} = \frac{\partial \mu}{\partial \theta}$. The function $V(\mu) = \frac{\partial \mu}{\partial \theta}$ is called the variance function. Hence, there is an explicit relation between the expected value and the variance of any exponential model: $\mathrm{var}(Y) = V(\mu)a(\phi)$.

The function $a(\phi)$ is often of the form $a(\phi) = \phi/\omega$, where ω is a weighting term. In this case, the parameter ϕ is known as the dispersion parameter.   □

Equation [2.2] is easy to show. Suppose that $\theta \mapsto \int f(y; \theta, \phi) dy$ is twice differentiable at every θ, and suppose further that we may swap the order of differentiation and integration, i.e.:

$$\int \frac{\partial^2}{\partial \theta^2} f(y; \theta, \phi)\, dy = \frac{\partial^2}{\partial \theta^2} \int f(y; \theta, \phi)\, dy.$$

Then:

$$\frac{\partial}{\partial \theta} f(y; \theta, \phi) = \left(\frac{y - \dot{b}(\theta)}{a(\phi)} \right) f(y; \theta, \phi),$$

and

$$\frac{\partial^2}{\partial \theta^2} f(y; \theta, \phi) = -\frac{\ddot{b}(\theta)}{a(\phi)} f(y; \theta, \phi) + \left(\frac{y - \dot{b}(\theta)}{a(\phi)} \right)^2 f(y; \theta, \phi).$$

Integrating both sides of these two equalities with respect to y gives:

$$0 = \mathbb{E}\left(\frac{Y - \dot{b}(\theta)}{a(\phi)} \right) \quad \text{and} \quad 0 = -\frac{\ddot{b}(\theta)}{a(\phi)} + \mathbb{E}\left[\left(\frac{Y - \dot{b}(\theta)}{a(\phi)} \right)^2 \right],$$

since

$$\int \frac{\partial}{\partial \theta} f(y; \theta, \phi)\, dy = \frac{\partial}{\partial \theta} \int f(y; \theta, \phi)\, dy = \frac{\partial}{\partial \theta} 1 = 0,$$

and

$$\int \frac{\partial^2}{\partial \theta^2} f(y; \theta, \phi) \, dy = \frac{\partial^2}{\partial \theta^2} \int f(y; \theta, \phi) \, dy = \frac{\partial^2}{\partial \theta^2} 1 = 0.$$

This gives us the expressions in equation [2.2].

2.1.2. Examples

This section lists some of the most significant examples of exponential families. Interested readers can find more examples in [DEJ 08, MCC 89].

EXAMPLE 2.1.– The family of Gaussian distributions $Y \sim \mathcal{N}(\mu, \sigma^2)$ with mean μ and variance σ^2 is an exponential family. The probability density function of Y is:

$$f(y) = \frac{1}{\sigma\sqrt{2\pi}} \exp\left(-\frac{1}{2\sigma^2}(y - \mu)^2\right), \quad y \in \mathbb{R},$$

$$= \exp\left(\frac{\mu y - \frac{\mu^2}{2}}{\sigma^2} - \frac{1}{2}\left[\ln(2\pi\sigma^2) + \frac{y^2}{\sigma^2}\right]\right),$$

which can be identified with the density function in equation [2.1] by setting $\theta = \mu$, $\phi = \sigma^2$, $a(\phi) = \phi$, $b(\theta) = \frac{\theta^2}{2}$ and $c(y, \phi) = -\frac{1}{2}\left[\ln(2\pi\sigma^2) + \frac{y^2}{\sigma^2}\right]$. It is easy to check that:

$$\mathbb{E}(Y) = \dot{b}(\theta) = \theta = \mu \quad \text{and} \quad \text{var}(Y) = \ddot{b}(\theta)a(\phi) = 1 \cdot \sigma^2 = \sigma^2.$$

Here, the variance function $V(\mu)$ is simply 1. □

EXAMPLE 2.2.– The family of binomial distributions $Y \sim \mathcal{B}(m, \pi)$ is another exponential family. The density function of Y is:

$$f(y) = C_m^y \pi^y (1 - \pi)^{m-y}, \quad y = 0, 1, \dots, m,$$

$$= \exp\left(y \ln\left(\frac{\pi}{1 - \pi}\right) + m \ln(1 - \pi) + \ln C_m^y\right),$$

which can be identified with equation [2.1] by setting $\theta = \ln(\frac{\pi}{1-\pi})$, $\phi = 1$, $a(\phi) = \phi$, $b(\theta) = -m \ln(1 - \pi) = m \ln(1 + e^\theta)$ and $c(y, \phi) = \ln C_m^y$. Again, it is easy to check that:

$$\mathbb{E}(Y) = \dot{b}(\theta) = m \frac{e^\theta}{1 + e^\theta} = m\pi$$

and

$$\text{var}(Y) = \ddot{b}(\theta)a(\phi) = m\frac{e^\theta}{1+e^\theta}\frac{1}{1+e^\theta} = m\pi(1-\pi).$$

Let $\mu = \mathbb{E}(Y) = m\pi$. The variance function $V(\mu)$ is given by $V(\mu) = \mu(m-\mu)/m$. □

REMARK.– The function from $]0,1[$ to $\mathbb{R}$ defined by $x \mapsto \ln(\frac{x}{1-x})$ is called the logistic function. It is sometimes written $\text{logit}(x) = \ln(\frac{x}{1-x})$. □

EXAMPLE 2.3.– The family of Poisson distributions $Y \sim \mathcal{P}(\mu)$ is also an exponential family. The density function of Y is:

$$f(y) = \exp(-\mu)\frac{\mu^y}{y!}, \quad y = 0,1,2,\ldots,$$

$$= \exp\left(-\mu + y\ln\mu - \ln y!\right),$$

which can be identified with equation [2.1] by setting $\theta = \ln\mu$, $\phi = 1$, $a(\phi) = \phi$, $b(\theta) = \mu = e^\theta$ and $c(y,\phi) = -\ln y!$. We note that:

$$\mathbb{E}(Y) = \dot{b}(\theta) = e^\theta = \mu \quad \text{and} \quad \text{var}(Y) = \ddot{b}(\theta)a(\phi) = e^\theta = \mu.$$

As expected, this recovers the equidispersion property of the Poisson distribution (the mean and variance are equal). Here, the variance function $V(\mu)$ is given by $V(\mu) = \mu$. □

EXAMPLE 2.4.– The family of gamma distributions $Y \sim G(\mu,\nu)$ is also an exponential family. There are multiple possible parameterizations of the gamma distribution. The benefit of the approach chosen here is that a simple expression is obtained for $\mathbb{E}(Y)$. With this parameterization, the density function of Y is[1]:

$$f(y) = y^{-1}\exp\left(-\frac{y\nu}{\mu}\right)\left(\frac{y\nu}{\mu}\right)^\nu\frac{1}{\Gamma(\nu)}, \quad y > 0,$$

$$= \exp\left(\frac{-\mu^{-1}y - \ln\mu}{\nu^{-1}} + (\nu-1)\ln y + \nu\ln\nu - \ln\Gamma(\nu)\right),$$

$$[2.3]$$

---

1 Recall that the gamma function is defined as $\Gamma : x \mapsto \int_0^{+\infty} e^{-t}t^{x-1}\,dt$.

which can be identified with equation [2.1] by setting $\theta = -1/\mu$, $\phi = 1/\nu$, $a(\phi) = \phi$, $b(\theta) = \ln \mu = -\ln(-\theta)$ and $c(y, \phi) = (\nu - 1) \ln y + \nu \ln \nu - \ln \Gamma(\nu)$. This time:

$$\mathbb{E}(Y) = \dot{b}(\theta) = -\frac{1}{\theta} = \mu \quad \text{and} \quad \text{var}(Y) = \ddot{b}(\theta)a(\phi) = \frac{\phi}{\theta^2} = \frac{\mu^2}{\nu}.$$

The variance function $V(\mu)$ is given by $V(\mu) = \mu^2$.   □

EXAMPLE 2.5.– The negative binomial distribution is defined as the probability distribution of the random variable Y representing the number of failures required before k successes are obtained (where $k \in \{1, 2, \ldots\}$) in a sequence of independent random trials with constant probability of success π. The probability density function of this distribution is:

$$f(y) = C_{y+k-1}^y \pi^k (1 - \pi)^y, \quad y = 0, 1, 2, \ldots$$

We recall that for any given integer n, $\Gamma(n + 1) = n!$. Let $\kappa = 1/k$ and $\mu = k\left(\frac{1-\pi}{\pi}\right)$. Then, f can be rewritten as:

$$f(y) = \frac{\Gamma(y + \frac{1}{\kappa})}{y!\Gamma(\frac{1}{\kappa})} \left(\frac{\kappa\mu}{1 + \kappa\mu}\right)^y \left(\frac{1}{1 + \kappa\mu}\right)^{\frac{1}{\kappa}}, \quad y = 0, 1, 2, \ldots \quad [2.4]$$

This expression makes it easier to see that the family of negative binomial distributions is an exponential family. The density function of Y is:

$$f(y) = \exp\left(y \ln\left(\frac{\kappa\mu}{1 + \kappa\mu}\right) - \frac{1}{\kappa} \ln(1 + \kappa\mu)\right.$$
$$\left. + \ln \Gamma\left(y + \frac{1}{\kappa}\right) - \ln\left(y!\Gamma\left(\frac{1}{\kappa}\right)\right)\right),$$

which can be identified with equation [2.1] by setting $\theta = \ln\left(\frac{\kappa\mu}{1+\kappa\mu}\right)$, $\phi = 1$, $a(\phi) = \phi$, $b(\theta) = \frac{1}{\kappa} \ln(1 + \kappa\mu) = -\frac{1}{\kappa} \ln(1 - e^\theta)$ and $c(y, \phi) = \ln \Gamma\left(y + \frac{1}{\kappa}\right) - \ln\left(y!\Gamma\left(\frac{1}{\kappa}\right)\right)$. The mean value and variance are:

$$\mathbb{E}(Y) = \dot{b}(\theta) = \frac{1}{\kappa}\frac{e^\theta}{1 - e^\theta} = \frac{1}{\kappa}\kappa\mu = \mu$$

and

$$\mathrm{var}(Y) = \ddot{b}(\theta)a(\phi) = \frac{1}{\kappa}\frac{e^{\theta}}{(1-e^{\theta})^2} = \mu(1+\kappa\mu).$$

The variance function $V(\mu)$ is given by $V(\mu) = \mu(1+\kappa\mu)$. □

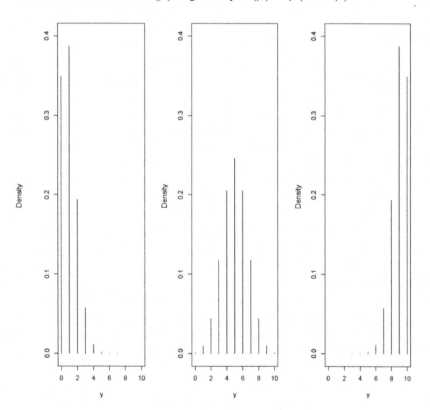

Figure 2.1. *Binomial distribution $\mathcal{B}(m,\pi)$ for $m = 10$ and $\pi = 0.1$ (left),*
$\pi = 0.5$ (center) and $\pi = 0.9$ (right)

The density functions of a few binomial, Poisson, gamma and negative binomial distributions are shown in Figures 2.1, 2.2, 2.3 and 2.4, respectively. The following R code [RCO 17] was used to generate Figure 2.1 and can easily be adapted for the other figures.

```
n=10; x=0:n; pi=c(0.1,0.5,0.9)

par(mfrow = c(1,3))
for (j in 1:3){
plot(x,dbinom(x,n,pi[j]),type="h",xlab="y",ylab="density"
    ,ylim=c(0,0.4))
}
```

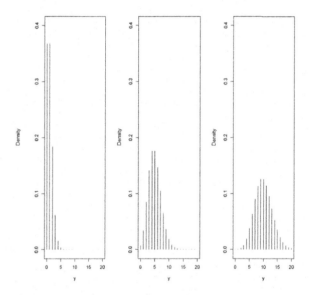

Figure 2.2. *Poisson distribution $\mathcal{P}(\mu)$ for $\mu = 1$ (left),
$\mu = 5$ (center) and $\mu = 10$ (right)*

REMARK.– For each of the examples above, the canonical parameter θ is a function of the expected value $\mu := \mathbb{E}(Y)$:

$$\theta = g(\mu).$$

This function g is known as the *canonical link function*. We note that $\mu = \mathbb{E}(Y) = \dot{b}(\theta)$ (by equation [2.2]), so $\theta = g(\dot{b}(\theta))$ and hence $g = \dot{b}^{-1}$.

For the Gaussian distribution $Y \sim \mathcal{N}(\mu, \sigma^2)$, $\theta = \mathrm{id}(\mu)$ (the "identity" link function). For the binomial distribution $Y \sim \mathcal{B}(m, \pi)$, $\theta = \ln(\frac{\pi}{1-\pi}) = \ln(\frac{\mu}{m-\mu})$ (the "logit" link function). For the Poisson distribution $Y \sim \mathcal{P}(\mu)$, $\theta = \ln \mu$ (the "log" link function). For the gamma distribution $Y \sim G(\mu, \nu)$, $\theta = -\frac{1}{\mu}$. For the negative binomial distribution, $\theta = \ln(\frac{\kappa\mu}{1+\kappa\mu})$. □

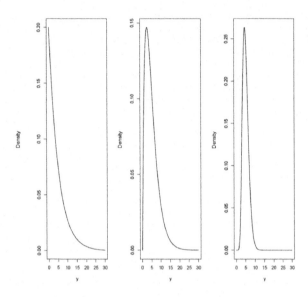

Figure 2.3. *Gamma distribution $G(\mu, \nu)$ for $\mu = 5$ and $\nu = 1$ (left), $\nu = 2$ (center) and $\nu = 10$ (right)*

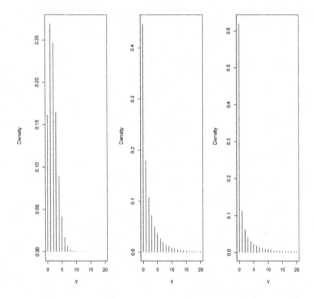

Figure 2.4. *Negative binomial distribution for $\mu = 2$ and $\kappa = 0.1$ (left), $\kappa = 2$ (center) and $\kappa = 5$ (right)*

Generalized linear models, first formalized by Nelder and Wedderburn [NEL 72], offer a general framework for describing the relationship between a response variable and a set of explanatory variables. The next few sections give a definition of generalized linear models and an overview of some of the principles of estimation associated with them. Interested readers can find a more in-depth discussion in [DOB 10, DEJ 08, MCC 89].

2.2. The components of a generalized linear model

To define a generalized linear model, we need three elements: a random component, a so-called systematic component and a link function.

2.2.1. *Random component*

The random component specifies the probability distribution of the response variable (or its conditional distribution given the explanatory variables if applicable). In the context of a generalized linear model, this distribution is assumed to belong to an exponential family.

Accordingly, we assume that the sample of observations is composed of n independent variables $Z_1, \ldots, Z_n$ and that the density function of each Z_i (with respect to the relevant dominating measure: the Lebesgue measure on $\mathbb{R}$ or the counting measure on $\mathbb{N}$) is of the form:

$$f(z_i; \theta_i, \phi) = \exp\left(\frac{\theta_i z_i - b(\theta_i)}{a(\phi)} + c(z_i, \phi)\right), \quad i = 1, \ldots, n,$$

where $a(\cdot)$, $b(\cdot)$ and $c(\cdot, \cdot)$ specify the model (e.g. binomial, Poisson). The dispersion parameter ϕ is assumed to be identical for every observation (in particular, it is simply 1 for the binomial, Poisson and negative binomial distributions). The most appropriate choice of distribution depends on the nature of the response variable (binary variable, count variable, continuous variable, etc.).

2.2.2. *Systematic component*

The systematic component is a linear combination $\beta^\top \mathbf{X}_i$ of the explanatory variables (using the same notation as for the linear model, i.e. $\mathbf{X}_i = (X_{i1}, X_{i2}, \ldots, X_{ip})^\top$ and $\beta = (\beta_1, \ldots, \beta_p)^\top)$. This linear combination can include functions of the original explanatory variables (e.g. $\ln X_{i2}$), as well as interactions (e.g. $X_{i2} \times X_{i3}$). The vector $\beta \in \mathbb{R}^p$ is a vector of unknowns.

2.2.3. Link function

The third component of the generalized linear model specifies the relation between the response variable Z_i and the linear predictor $\beta^\top \mathbf{X}_i$. Let $\mu_i = \mathbb{E}(Z_i | \mathbf{X}_i)$, and we define:

$$g(\mu_i) = \beta^\top \mathbf{X}_i, \quad i = 1, \ldots, n,$$

where g is a monotonic and differentiable function, known as the link function. The canonical link function $g = \dot{b}^{-1}$ is often used. In this case, $\theta_i = g(\mu_i) = \beta^\top \mathbf{X}_i$.

REMARK.– Let Z_i, $i = 1, \ldots, n$, be independent observations from $\mathcal{N}(\beta^\top \mathbf{X}_i, \sigma^2)$. As shown in Example 2.1, the density function of Z_i is indeed of the form of equation [2.1], with $\theta_i = \beta^\top \mathbf{X}_i$. Here, $\mu_i = \mathbb{E}(Z_i) = \theta_i = \beta^\top \mathbf{X}_i$ (the link function is the identity).

This model is equivalent to the Gaussian linear model, which is more commonly presented in the form:

$$Z_i = \beta^\top \mathbf{X}_i + \epsilon_i, \quad \epsilon_i \overset{i.i.d.}{\sim} \mathcal{N}(0, \sigma^2), \quad i = 1, \ldots, n.$$

The Gaussian linear model is therefore a generalized linear model. □

2.3. Maximum likelihood estimator

2.3.1. Likelihood equations

To estimate the parameters of a generalized linear model, we use the maximum likelihood method. Suppose that we have a sample $Z_1, \ldots, Z_n$ of independent observations with density functions:

$$f(z_i; \theta_i, \phi) = \exp\left(\frac{\theta_i z_i - b(\theta_i)}{a(\phi)} + c(z_i, \phi)\right), \quad i = 1, \ldots, n.$$

For each individual i, we also have a vector $\mathbf{X}_i = (X_{i1}, X_{i2}, \ldots, X_{ip})^\top$ of explanatory variables (which can be either quantitative or qualitative).

We recall the following notations: $\mu_i = \mathbb{E}(Z_i|\mathbf{X}_i)$ denotes the expected value of Z_i given the covariables, and $g(\mu_i) = \beta^\top \mathbf{X}_i$ is the link function (which may or may not be the canonical link function). In the following, we will also write $\eta_i = \beta^\top \mathbf{X}_i$.

Let us compute the likelihood of the parameter (β, ϕ) with respect to the independent sample $(Z_1, \mathbf{X}_1), \ldots, (Z_n, \mathbf{X}_n)$:

$$L_n(\beta, \phi) = \prod_{i=1}^n \exp\left(\frac{\theta_i Z_i - b(\theta_i)}{a(\phi)} + c(Z_i, \phi) \right).$$

This gives us the log-likelihood $\ell_n(\beta, \phi) = \ln L_n(\beta, \phi)$:

$$\ell_n(\beta, \phi) = \sum_{i=1}^n \left\{ \frac{\theta_i Z_i - b(\theta_i)}{a(\phi)} + c(Z_i, \phi) \right\} := \sum_{i=1}^n \ell_{n,i}(\beta, \phi).$$

The maximum likelihood estimator $\hat{\beta}_n$ of β is obtained by solving the equation (here, the system of p equations):

$$\frac{\partial}{\partial \beta} \ell_n(\beta, \phi) \Big|_{\beta = \hat{\beta}_n} = \sum_{i=1}^n \frac{\partial}{\partial \beta} \ell_{n,i}(\beta, \phi) \Big|_{\beta = \hat{\beta}_n} = 0.$$

For each $j = 1, \ldots, p$:

$$\frac{\partial \ell_{n,i}}{\partial \beta_j} = \frac{\partial \ell_{n,i}}{\partial \theta_i} \frac{\partial \theta_i}{\partial \mu_i} \frac{\partial \mu_i}{\partial \eta_i} \frac{\partial \eta_i}{\partial \beta_j}.$$

REMARK.– We will use "Leibniz" notation for the derivatives of composite functions: if $z = f(y)$ and $y = g(x)$, then the derivative $\partial f(g(x))/\partial x = \dot{f}(g(x))\dot{g}(x)$ is written as $\frac{\partial z}{\partial x} = \frac{\partial z}{\partial y} \frac{\partial y}{\partial x}$. □

We have that:

$$\frac{\partial \ell_{n,i}}{\partial \theta_i} = \frac{Z_i - \dot{b}(\theta_i)}{a(\phi)} = \frac{Z_i - \mu_i}{a(\phi)}$$

$$\frac{\partial \mu_i}{\partial \theta_i} = V(\mu_i) = \frac{\text{var}(Z_i)}{a(\phi)}$$

$$\frac{\partial \eta_i}{\partial \beta_j} = X_{ij}.$$

By contrast, the term $\partial \mu_i / \partial \eta_i$ depends on the choice of link function $g(\mu_i) = \eta_i$:

$$\frac{\partial}{\partial \beta_j} \ell_n(\beta, \phi) = \sum_{i=1}^{n} X_{ij} \frac{(Z_i - \mu_i)}{V(\mu_i) a(\phi)} \frac{\partial \mu_i}{\partial \eta_i}, \quad j = 1, \ldots, p. \qquad [2.5]$$

This gives us the estimation equations (also known as the score equations or the likelihood equations) of the parameters β_j:

$$\sum_{i=1}^{n} X_{ij} \frac{(Z_i - \mu_i)}{V(\mu_i)} \frac{\partial \mu_i}{\partial \eta_i} = 0, \quad j = 1, \ldots, p. \qquad [2.6]$$

These equations are nonlinear in β (except in certain special cases, such as Example 2.1) and usually cannot be solved analytically. We will use iterative algorithms (e.g. the Newton–Raphson algorithm or the Fisher scoring algorithm) to approximate the maximum likelihood estimator (see section 2.3.4).

REMARK.– Equation [2.6] depends on β via the terms μ_i and η_i, $i = 1, \ldots, n$ (although this dependence was omitted to simplify the notation). However, it does not depend on ϕ and therefore neither does the maximum likelihood estimator of β. The parameter ϕ can be estimated separately (see section 2.3.5). $\qquad \square$

2.3.2. *Case of a canonical link function*

Suppose that g is chosen as the canonical link function. In this case, $\theta_i = g(\mu_i) = \beta^\top \mathbf{X}_i = \eta_i$, and the likelihood equations simplify. We have that:

$$\frac{\partial \mu_i}{\partial \eta_i} = \frac{\partial \mu_i}{\partial \theta_i} = V(\mu_i),$$

and equation [2.6] now reduces to:

$$\sum_{i=1}^{n} X_{ij}(Z_i - \mu_i) = 0, \quad j = 1, \dots, p. \tag{2.7}$$

These p equations can also be written in matrix form. As in section 1.3, the design matrix is defined as:

$$\mathbb{X} = \begin{pmatrix} 1 & X_{12} & \cdots & X_{1p} \\ 1 & X_{22} & \cdots & X_{2p} \\ \vdots & \vdots & \ddots & \vdots \\ 1 & X_{n2} & \cdots & X_{np} \end{pmatrix},$$

where the i-th row ($i = 1, \dots, n$) contains the explanatory variables of the i-th individual and the j-th column ($j = 1, \dots, p$) contains the values of the j-th variable on each of the n individuals. Below, we will assume that $\mathbb{X}$ has rank p.

Next, let $\mathbf{Z} = (Z_1, \dots, Z_n)^\top$ and $\mu = (\mu_1, \dots, \mu_n)^\top$. We can write the system of p equations from equation [2.7] in the form:

$$\mathbb{X}^\top (\mathbf{Z} - \mu) = 0. \tag{2.8}$$

EXAMPLE 2.6.– Consider a Gaussian linear model. In this case, $\mu_i = \beta^\top \mathbf{X}_i$ and $\mu = \mathbb{X}\beta$. Equation [2.8] becomes:

$$\mathbb{X}^\top (\mathbf{Z} - \mathbb{X}\beta) = 0.$$

The solution of this equation is $\hat{\beta}_n = (\mathbb{X}^\top \mathbb{X})^{-1} \mathbb{X}^\top \mathbf{Z}$ whenever $\mathbb{X}^\top \mathbb{X}$ is invertible. Thus, we recover the maximum likelihood estimator of β stated earlier for the Gaussian linear model. □

EXAMPLE 2.7.– Let Z_i follow a binomial distribution $\mathcal{B}(m_i, p(\mathbf{X}_i))$, so that $\mu_i = \mathbb{E}(Z_i|\mathbf{X}_i) = m_i p(\mathbf{X}_i)$. If g is the canonical link function, then:

$$g(\mu_i) = \ln\left(\frac{\mu_i}{m_i - \mu_i}\right) = \ln\left(\frac{p(\mathbf{X}_i)}{1 - p(\mathbf{X}_i)}\right) = \text{logit}(p(\mathbf{X}_i)) = \beta^\top \mathbf{X}_i.$$

In other words, $p(\mathbf{X}_i) = e^{\beta^\top \mathbf{X}_i}/(1 + e^{\beta^\top \mathbf{X}_i})$. The score equations for estimating β_j, $j = 1, \ldots, p$ are given by:

$$\sum_{i=1}^{n} X_{ij}(Z_i - m_i p(\mathbf{X}_i)) = 0, \quad j = 1, \ldots, p. \qquad [2.9]$$

Alternatively, in matrix form, $\mathbb{X}^\top(\mathbf{Z} - \mu) = 0$, where $\mu = (m_1 p(\mathbf{X}_1), \ldots, m_n p(\mathbf{X}_n))^\top$. In this case, the maximum likelihood estimator does not have an explicit expression and needs to be approximated numerically. □

EXAMPLE 2.8.– If Z_i follows a Poisson distribution $\mathcal{P}(\lambda(\mathbf{X}_i))$, then $\mu_i = \mathbb{E}(Z_i|\mathbf{X}_i) = \lambda(\mathbf{X}_i)$. If g is the canonical link function, then:

$$g(\mu_i) = \ln \mu_i = \ln \lambda(\mathbf{X}_i) = \beta^\top \mathbf{X}_i.$$

In other words, $\mu_i = \lambda(\mathbf{X}_i) = e^{\beta^\top \mathbf{X}_i}$. The score equations are given by:

$$\sum_{i=1}^{n} X_{ij}(Z_i - e^{\beta^\top \mathbf{X}_i}) = 0, \quad j = 1, \ldots, p. \qquad [2.10]$$

In matrix form, $\mathbb{X}^\top(\mathbf{Z} - \mu) = 0$, where $\mu = (e^{\beta^\top \mathbf{X}_1}, \ldots, e^{\beta^\top \mathbf{X}_n})^\top$. Again, the maximum likelihood estimator does not have an explicit expression and needs to be approximated numerically. □

EXAMPLE 2.9.– If Z_i follows a gamma distribution $G(\mu(\mathbf{X}_i), \nu)$, then $\mu_i = \mathbb{E}(Z_i|\mathbf{X}_i) = \mu(\mathbf{X}_i)$. If g is the canonical link function, then:

$$g(\mu_i) = -\frac{1}{\mu_i} = \beta^\top \mathbf{X}_i.$$

In other words, $\mu_i = -1/\beta^\top \mathbf{X}_i$. The support of the gamma distribution is $]0, \infty[$, so $\mu_i > 0$. Therefore, $\beta^\top \mathbf{X}_i < 0$, which restricts the estimates of β. Accordingly, the log link function is usually preferred:

$$\ln \mu_i = \beta^\top \mathbf{X}_i.$$

In other words, $\mu_i = e^{\beta^\top \mathbf{X}_i}$. In R, there are three choices of link function for the gamma distribution: the identity link function, the log link function and the inverse link function (defined by $g(\mu_i) = 1/\mu_i$). This "inverse" link function and the canonical link function are equivalent. To see this, we note that if $-1/\mu_i = \beta^\top \mathbf{X}_i$, then $1/\mu_i = \beta^{*\top} \mathbf{X}_i$, where $\beta^* = -\beta$.   □

REMARK.– In section 3.3, we will see that the log link function is also typically preferred over the canonical link function in the case of the negative binomial distribution.   □

2.3.3. *Asymptotic properties and inference*

In the context of a generalized linear model, statistical inference is performed by arguing from the asymptotic properties (consistency, asymptotic normality) of the maximum likelihood estimator. These properties were first established for the logistic model by [GOU 81]. They were shown to hold for arbitrary generalized linear models by [FAH 85] (either with the canonical link function or an arbitrary link function). An overview of the theorems stated below can be found in [ANT 92].

The following theorem (see [ANT 92]) gives sufficient conditions for the consistency and asymptotic normality of the maximum likelihood estimator $\hat{\beta}_n$ of a generalized linear model with a canonical link function. To simplify the notation, we assume that the dispersion parameter is known, and we write $\ell_n(\beta)$ for the log-likelihood. We will also write β for the true value of the parameter and $\mathcal{I}_n(\beta) = -\partial^2 \ell_n(\beta)/\partial\beta\partial\beta^\top$.

THEOREM.–   Given a generalized linear model, suppose that: i) the explanatory variables $X_{i1}, X_{i2}, \ldots, X_{ip}$ are bounded and ii) the smallest eigenvalue of the matrix $\mathbb{X}^\top \mathbb{X}$ tends to infinity as n tends to infinity. Then, the sequence $(\hat{\beta}_n)$ of maximum likelihood estimators converges in probability to β and $\mathcal{I}_n(\hat{\beta}_n)^{\frac{1}{2}}(\hat{\beta}_n - \beta)$ converges in distribution to the Gaussian vector $\mathcal{N}(0, I_p)$.

REMARK.– In section 1.6 (on the asymptotics of linear models), we noted that a condition for the maximum likelihood estimator to be consistent is for $(\mathbb{X}^\top \mathbb{X})^{-1}$ to converge to 0 as n tends to infinity.

This condition can be interpreted as stating that the information provided by the explanatory variables must continue to increase with n. Hypothesis ii) plays a similar role for generalized linear models. □

After fitting a model, we often need to find confidence intervals or regions for our parameters or test the significance of one or several regressors. Some examples of the most widely used confidence regions and hypothesis tests are given below.

2.3.3.1. *Confidence intervals and regions*

By the previous theorem, when n is large, the distribution of $\hat{\beta}_n$ is approximated by the Gaussian vector $\mathcal{N}(\beta, \mathcal{I}_n(\hat{\beta}_n)^{-1})$. If we write $\hat{\sigma}_j^2$ for the j-th term on the diagonal of $\mathcal{I}_n(\hat{\beta}_n)^{-1}$ and $\hat{\beta}_{n,j}$ for the j-th component of $\hat{\beta}_n$ (for $j = 1, \ldots, p$), then the distribution of $\hat{\beta}_{n,j}$ is approximated by the normal distribution $\mathcal{N}(\beta_j, \hat{\sigma}_j^2)$.

This gives a confidence interval with an asymptotic confidence level of $(1 - \alpha)$ for the parameter β_j:

$$\left[\hat{\beta}_{n,j} - u_{1-\alpha/2}\hat{\sigma}_j \; ; \hat{\beta}_{n,j} + u_{1-\alpha/2}\hat{\sigma}_j\right],$$

where $u_{1-\alpha/2}$ denotes the quantile of order $1 - \alpha/2$ of $\mathcal{N}(0,1)$, defined by $\mathbb{P}(\mathcal{N}(0,1) \leq u_{1-\alpha/2}) = 1 - \alpha/2$ (for $\alpha \in {]0,1[}$).

REMARK.– As for the linear model, the quantity $\hat{\sigma}_j$ (estimate of the asymptotic standard deviation of the estimator $\hat{\beta}_{n,j}$) is usually called the "standard error". □

The theorem also implies that $(\hat{\beta}_n - \beta)^\top \mathcal{I}_n(\hat{\beta}_n)(\hat{\beta}_n - \beta)$ converges in distribution to χ_p^2. This allows us to construct a confidence region to an asymptotic confidence level of $(1 - \alpha)$ for the parameter $\beta = (\beta_1, \ldots, \beta_p)^\top$. This confidence region is given by the set of values β for which:

$$(\hat{\beta}_n - \beta)^\top \mathcal{I}_n(\hat{\beta}_n)(\hat{\beta}_n - \beta) \leq c_p(1 - \alpha),$$

where $c_p(1 - \alpha)$ denotes the quantile of order $1 - \alpha$ of the distribution χ_p^2.

2.3.3.2. *Test for a single component of β (Wald test)*

Suppose that we wish to test the non-significance of the j-th explanatory variable of the linear predictor $\beta^\top \mathbf{X}_i$. In other words, we want to test the hypothesis $H_0 : \beta_j = 0$ against $H_1 : \beta_j \neq 0$. Under H_0, the Wald statistic $\hat{\beta}_{n,j}/\hat{\sigma}_j$ converges in distribution to $\mathcal{N}(0,1)$. We can therefore define the following region of rejection for H_0 to the asymptotic significance level of α:

$$\mathcal{R}_\alpha = \left\{ \left| \frac{\hat{\beta}_{n,j}}{\hat{\sigma}_j} \right| \geq u_{1-\alpha/2} \right\} .$$

2.3.3.3. *Likelihood-ratio test*

Suppose that we wish to test the simultaneous nullity of q parameters (without loss of generality, to simplify the notation, we can suppose that we are testing the nullity of the first q coefficients of β). The test problem may be stated as:

$$H_0 : \beta_1 = \ldots = \beta_q = 0$$

against

$$H_1 : \text{there exists } i \in \{1, \ldots, q\} \text{ such that } \beta_i \neq 0.$$

In practice, the most widely used test for this problem is the likelihood-ratio test. Intuitively, the likelihood-ratio test compares the likelihoods under H_0 and H_1 and accepts H_0 if they are "close". The likelihood under H_0 is $L_n(\hat{\beta}_{n,H_0})$, where $\hat{\beta}_{n,H_0}$ denotes the maximum likelihood estimator obtained with the constraint $\beta_1 = \ldots = \beta_q = 0$ (i.e. by eliminating the first q explanatory variables from the model). If H_0 holds, then $L_n(\hat{\beta}_{n,H_0})$ should be "close" to the maximum likelihood $L_n(\hat{\beta}_n)$ (the same reasoning can of course be applied to the log-likelihood). We therefore define the test statistic:

$$D_n = 2 \ln \left(\frac{L_n(\hat{\beta}_n)}{L_n(\hat{\beta}_{n,H_0})} \right) = 2(\ell_n(\hat{\beta}_n) - \ell_n(\hat{\beta}_{n,H_0})). \qquad [2.11]$$

If H_0 holds, it can be shown that D_n converges in distribution to the distribution χ^2_q as n tends to infinity. This gives us a region of rejection for H_0 to an asymptotic significance level of α:

$$\mathcal{R}^D_\alpha = \{D_n \geq c_q(1 - \alpha)\},$$

where $c_q(1 - \alpha)$ denotes the quantile of order $1 - \alpha$ of the distribution χ_q^2.

REMARK.– We could also use a Wald test to test H_0 against H_1. Let $\hat{\beta}_{n,1:q}$ be the vector composed of the first q components of $\hat{\beta}_n$ and let $M_q(\hat{\beta}_n)$ be the $q \times q$ submatrix containing the first q rows and columns of $(\mathcal{I}_n(\hat{\beta}_n))^{-1}$. Under H_0, the Wald statistic:

$$W_n = \hat{\beta}_{n,1:q}^\top M_q(\hat{\beta}_n)^{-1} \hat{\beta}_{n,1:q}$$

follows the asymptotic distribution χ_q^2. This allows us to deduce a region of rejection for H_0 to an asymptotic confidence level of α: $\mathcal{R}_\alpha^W = \{W_n \geq c_q(1 - \alpha)\}$. A third asymptotic test, known as the score test, can also be used. The score test is presented by [ANT 92]. □

2.3.3.4. Deviance

Consider the generalized linear model $\mathcal{M}$ defined by $g(\mu_i) = \beta^\top \mathbf{X}_i$. The deviance is defined as the distance between the log-likelihood values obtained from this model and a model that only assumes that $\mu_i = \mathbb{E}(Z_i|\mathbf{X}_i)$, $i = 1, \dots, n$. The latter model, known as the "saturated model", has one parameter μ_i for each individual i.

Let $\hat{\mu} = (\hat{\mu}_1, \dots, \hat{\mu}_n)$ be the maximum likelihood estimators of the μ_i in the saturated model and let $\hat{\beta}_n$ be the maximum likelihood estimator of β in the model $\mathcal{M}$. The deviance of $\mathcal{M}$ is defined by:

$$\text{dev}(\mathcal{M}) = 2(\ell_n(\hat{\mu}) - \ell_n(\hat{\beta}_n)).$$

This quantity can be interpreted as a measure of the goodness of fit of the model $\mathcal{M}$ with respect to a certain data set (relative to the saturated model, which perfectly fits to the data; we note however that the saturated model is useless in practice: it has one parameter for each individual in the sample and therefore does not provide any information about the effect of the explanatory variables on the response).

EXAMPLE 2.10.– Consider the binomial model $Z_i \sim \mathcal{B}(m_i, p_\beta(\mathbf{X}_i))$, where $\text{logit}(p_\beta(\mathbf{X}_i)) = \beta^\top \mathbf{X}_i$. Let $\mu_i(\beta) = \mathbb{E}(Z_i|\mathbf{X}_i) = m_i p_\beta(\mathbf{X}_i)$, and let $Z_i \sim \mathcal{B}(m_i, p_i)$, $i = 1, \dots, n$ be the saturated model, with $p_i \in]0, 1[$ and

$\mu_i = \mathbb{E}(Z_i) = m_i p_i$. The likelihood of $\mu = (\mu_1, \ldots, \mu_n)$ in this model can now be written as:

$$L_n(\mu) = \prod_{i=1}^{n} C_{m_i}^{Z_i} p_i^{Z_i} (1 - p_i)^{m_i - Z_i},$$

which gives us the log-likelihood:

$$\ell_n(\mu) = \sum_{i=1}^{n} \left\{ Z_i \ln p_i + (m_i - Z_i) \ln(1 - p_i) + \ln C_{m_i}^{Z_i} \right\},$$

and the score equations:

$$\frac{\partial \ell_n(\mu)}{\partial p_\ell} = \frac{Z_\ell}{p_\ell} - \frac{m_\ell - Z_\ell}{1 - p_\ell} = 0, \quad \ell = 1, \ldots, n.$$

Finally, we deduce the maximum likelihood estimator of p_ℓ:

$$\hat{p}_\ell = \frac{Z_\ell}{m_\ell}, \quad \ell = 1, \ldots, n,$$

as well as the maximum likelihood estimator of μ_ℓ:

$$\hat{\mu}_\ell = m_\ell \hat{p}_\ell = Z_\ell, \quad \ell = 1, \ldots, n.$$

We write $\mu_i(\hat{\beta}_n) = m_i p_{\hat{\beta}_n}(\mathbf{X}_i)$ for the maximum likelihood estimator of $\mu_i(\beta)$ and $\hat{\mu} = (\hat{\mu}_1, \ldots, \hat{\mu}_n)$. The deviance of the model $Z_i \sim \mathcal{B}(m_i, p_\beta(\mathbf{X}_i))$ is calculated as follows:

$$\text{dev} = 2(\ell_n(\hat{\mu}) - \ell_n(\hat{\beta}_n))$$

$$= 2 \sum_{i=1}^{n} \left\{ Z_i \ln \left(\frac{Z_i}{m_i p_{\hat{\beta}_n}(\mathbf{X}_i)} \right) + (m_i - Z_i) \ln \left(\frac{m_i - Z_i}{m_i - m_i p_{\hat{\beta}_n}(\mathbf{X}_i)} \right) \right\}$$

$$= 2 \sum_{i=1}^{n} \left\{ Z_i \ln \left(\frac{Z_i}{\mu_i(\hat{\beta}_n)} \right) + (m_i - Z_i) \ln \left(\frac{m_i - Z_i}{m_i - \mu_i(\hat{\beta}_n)} \right) \right\}. \qquad \square$$

EXAMPLE 2.11.– Consider the Poisson model $Z_i \sim \mathcal{P}(\lambda(\mathbf{X}_i))$, where $\lambda(\mathbf{X}_i) = \exp(\beta^\top \mathbf{X}_i)$. Let $\mu_i(\beta) = \mathbb{E}(Z_i|\mathbf{X}_i) = \lambda(\mathbf{X}_i)$, and let $Z_i \sim \mathcal{P}(\lambda_i)$, $i = 1, \dots, n$ be the saturated model, with $\lambda_i > 0$ and $\mu_i = \mathbb{E}(Z_i) = \lambda_i$. The likelihood of $\mu = (\mu_1, \dots, \mu_n)$ is:

$$L_n(\mu) = \prod_{i=1}^{n} e^{-\lambda_i} \frac{\lambda_i^{Z_i}}{Z_i!},$$

which gives us the log-likelihood:

$$\ell_n(\mu) = \sum_{i=1}^{n} \{Z_i \ln \lambda_i - \lambda_i - \ln(Z_i!)\},$$

and the score equations:

$$\frac{\partial \ell_n(\mu)}{\partial \lambda_\ell} = \frac{Z_\ell}{\lambda_\ell} - 1 = 0, \quad \ell = 1, \dots, n.$$

Finally, the maximum likelihood estimator of μ_ℓ is:

$$\hat{\mu}_\ell = \hat{\lambda}_\ell = Z_\ell, \quad \ell = 1, \dots, n.$$

Let $\mu_i(\hat{\beta}_n) = \exp(\hat{\beta}_n^\top \mathbf{X}_i)$ be the maximum likelihood estimator of $\mu_i(\beta)$. The deviance is given by:

$$\text{dev} = 2 \sum_{i=1}^{n} \left\{ Z_i \ln \left(\frac{Z_i}{\mu_i(\hat{\beta}_n)} \right) - (Z_i - \mu_i(\hat{\beta}_n)) \right\}. \qquad \Box$$

We consider again the test problem:

$H_0 : \beta_1 = \dots = \beta_q = 0$

against

$H_1 :$ there exists $i \in \{1, \dots, q\}$ such that $\beta_i \neq 0$.

Let $\text{dev}(\mathcal{M}_{H_0})$ and $\text{dev}(\mathcal{M}_{H_1})$ be the deviance of the models obtained by assuming H_0 and H_1, respectively. Then, the test statistic in equation [2.11] satisfies:

$$
\begin{aligned}
D_n &= 2(\ell_n(\hat{\beta}_n) - \ell_n(\hat{\beta}_{n,H_0})) \\
&= 2(\ell_n(\hat{\mu}) - \ell_n(\hat{\beta}_{n,H_0})) - 2(\ell_n(\hat{\mu}) - \ell_n(\hat{\beta}_n)) \\
&= \text{dev}(\mathcal{M}_{H_0}) - \text{dev}(\mathcal{M}_{H_1}).
\end{aligned}
$$

The likelihood-ratio test compares the likelihood of the models under H_0 and H_1 (or, equivalently, their deviance). For this reason, it is sometimes called the deviance test.

2.3.4. Newton–Raphson algorithm

Except in some special cases, the maximum likelihood estimator of β in a generalized linear model does not have an explicit expression. Instead, we need to approximate it numerically using iterative algorithms such as the Newton–Raphson algorithm. The principles of this algorithm are outlined below.

The objective is to solve the likelihood equation:

$$
\frac{\partial \ell_n(\hat{\beta}_n)}{\partial \beta} := \frac{\partial}{\partial \beta} \ell_n(\beta) \bigg|_{\beta = \hat{\beta}_n} = 0.
$$

We recall that the solution of this equation does not depend on ϕ; hence, we will simply write $\ell_n(\beta)$ rather than $\ell_n(\beta, \phi)$ below. We will approximate the function $\partial \ell_n(\beta)/\partial \beta$ by its first-order Taylor expansion. Writing $\beta^{(i)}$ for the approximation of $\hat{\beta}_n$ obtained after the i-th iteration of the algorithm, we need to find $\beta^{(i+1)}$ such that:

$$
0 = \frac{\partial \ell_n(\beta^{(i+1)})}{\partial \beta} = \frac{\partial \ell_n(\beta^{(i)})}{\partial \beta} + \frac{\partial^2 \ell_n(\beta^{(i)})}{\partial \beta \partial \beta^{\top}} (\beta^{(i+1)} - \beta^{(i)}).
$$

This gives:

$$
\beta^{(i+1)} = \beta^{(i)} - \left(\frac{\partial^2 \ell_n(\beta^{(i)})}{\partial \beta \partial \beta^{\top}} \right)^{-1} \frac{\partial \ell_n(\beta^{(i)})}{\partial \beta}. \tag{2.12}
$$

The expression of $\partial \ell_n(\beta)/\partial \beta_j$ follows from equation [2.5]. The value of $\partial^2 \ell_n(\beta)/\partial \beta \partial \beta^\top$ is computed in a technical appendix at the end of this section.

Starting from some initial value $\beta^{(0)}$, equation [2.12] is iterated until a convergence criterion is satisfied (e.g. when the norm $\|\beta^{(i+1)} - \beta^{(i)}\|$ of the difference between two consecutive iterations is smaller than a fixed threshold $\varepsilon > 0$).

Case of a canonical link function

When the link function is the canonical link function, equation [2.12] simplifies:

$$\frac{\partial \ell_n(\beta)}{\partial \beta} = \frac{1}{a(\phi)} \mathbb{X}^\top (\mathbf{Z} - \mu(\beta)) \quad \text{and}$$

$$\frac{\partial^2 \ell_n(\beta)}{\partial \beta \partial \beta^\top} = -\frac{1}{a(\phi)} \mathbb{X}^\top W(\beta) \mathbb{X}, \tag{2.13}$$

where $\mu(\beta) = (\mu_1(\beta), \ldots, \mu_n(\beta))^\top$ and $W(\beta)$ denotes the diagonal matrix with j-th diagonal term $V(\mu_j(\beta))$, $j = 1, \ldots, n$. Equation [2.12] therefore becomes:

$$\beta^{(i+1)} = \beta^{(i)} + (\mathbb{X}^\top W(\beta^{(i)}) \mathbb{X})^{-1} \mathbb{X}^\top (\mathbf{Z} - \mu(\beta^{(i)}))$$

$$= (\mathbb{X}^\top W(\beta^{(i)}) \mathbb{X})^{-1} \left[\mathbb{X}^\top W(\beta^{(i)}) \mathbb{X} \beta^{(i)} + \mathbb{X}^\top (\mathbf{Z} - \mu(\beta^{(i)})) \right]$$

$$= (\mathbb{X}^\top W(\beta^{(i)}) \mathbb{X})^{-1} \mathbb{X}^\top W(\beta^{(i)}) \left[\mathbb{X} \beta^{(i)} + W(\beta^{(i)})^{-1} (\mathbf{Z} - \mu(\beta^{(i)})) \right]$$

$$= (\mathbb{X}^\top W(\beta^{(i)}) \mathbb{X})^{-1} \mathbb{X}^\top W(\beta^{(i)}) \mathbf{U}(\beta^{(i)}),$$

where $\mathbf{U}(\beta^{(i)}) := \mathbb{X} \beta^{(i)} + W(\beta^{(i)})^{-1} (\mathbf{Z} - \mu(\beta^{(i)}))$. Thus, at the $(i+1)$-th iteration of the algorithm, $\beta^{(i+1)}$ has the expression:

$$\beta^{(i+1)} \equiv (\mathbb{X}^\top W \mathbb{X})^{-1} \mathbb{X}^\top W \mathbf{U}, \tag{2.14}$$

which is of the form of a least squares estimator weighted by W (the vector $\mathbf{U}$ plays the role of a response variable and $\mathbb{X}$ is the design matrix). We note that W and $\mathbf{U}$ are updated at each iteration of the algorithm, since they depend on $\beta^{(i)}$.

Equation [2.14] illustrates why this algorithm is sometimes called the iteratively reweighted least squares algorithm.

REMARK.– In the Gaussian linear model, $V(\mu_j(\beta)) = 1$ for all $j = 1, \ldots, n$, and so $W(\beta)$ is the identity matrix of size n. Furthermore, $\mu(\beta) = \mathbb{X}\beta$, and so $U(\beta) = \mathbb{X}\beta + Z - \mathbb{X}\beta = Z$, which is independent of the iteration i. Hence, we recover the explicit solution $(\mathbb{X}^\top\mathbb{X})^{-1}\mathbb{X}^\top Z$ of the likelihood equation.   □

In R, generalized linear models are implemented by the glm function from the stats package.

The glm function uses a modified version of the Newton–Raphson algorithm, known as the Fischer scoring algorithm, which is often more efficient than the original Newton–Raphson algorithm. In the Fisher-scoring algorithm, $\mathcal{I}_n(\beta) = -\partial^2\ell_n(\beta)/\partial\beta\partial\beta^\top$ is replaced by $\mathbb{E}[\mathcal{I}_n(\beta)]$ in equation [2.12]. The matrix $\mathcal{I}_n(\beta)$ is often called the "observed information matrix", and $\mathbb{E}[\mathcal{I}_n(\beta)]$ is similarly known as the "expected information matrix."

REMARK.– In equation [2.13], in the case of a canonical link function, we note that the matrices $\mathcal{I}_n(\beta)$ and $\mathbb{E}[\mathcal{I}_n(\beta)]$ are identical. Accordingly, the Newton–Raphson and Fisher-scoring algorithms are also identical.   □

2.3.5. *Estimation of the dispersion parameter*

If the dispersion parameter ϕ is not known, then we need to estimate it. We recall that $\text{var}(Y) = V(\mu)a(\phi)$, where $V(\mu)$ is the variance function. We consider the case where $a(\phi) = \phi$. Then:

$$\phi = \frac{\text{var}(Y)}{V(\mu)},$$

where $g(\mu) = \beta^\top X$. There are several possible choices of estimator for ϕ. One of the most widely used is Pearson's χ^2 estimator, which is a moment-type estimator defined by:

$$\hat{\phi} = \frac{1}{n-p}\sum_{i=1}^{n}\frac{(Y_i - \hat{\mu}_i)^2}{V(\hat{\mu}_i)},$$

where $\hat{\mu}_i = g^{-1}(\hat{\beta}_n^\top X_i)$.

2.3.6. *Technical appendix*

We recall the formula from equation [2.5]:

$$\frac{\partial \ell_n(\beta)}{\partial \beta_j} = \sum_{i=1}^{n} X_{ij} \frac{(Z_i - \mu_i)}{V(\mu_i)a(\phi)} \frac{\partial \mu_i}{\partial \eta_i}$$

$$= \sum_{i=1}^{n} s_{i,j}(\beta, \phi), \quad j = 1, \ldots, p.$$

Let us now compute:

$$\frac{\partial^2 \ell_n(\beta)}{\partial \beta_j \partial \beta_k} = \sum_{i=1}^{n} \frac{\partial s_{i,j}(\beta, \phi)}{\partial \beta_k}, \quad j, k = 1, \ldots, p.$$

We have:

$$\frac{\partial s_{i,j}}{\partial \beta_k} = \frac{\partial s_{i,j}}{\partial \mu_i} \frac{\partial \mu_i}{\partial \eta_i} \frac{\partial \eta_i}{\partial \beta_k},$$

where

$$\frac{\partial s_{i,j}}{\partial \mu_i} = X_{ij} \frac{\partial}{\partial \mu_i} \left[\frac{(Z_i - \mu_i)}{V(\mu_i)a(\phi)} \frac{\partial \mu_i}{\partial \eta_i} \right] \quad \text{and} \quad \frac{\partial \eta_i}{\partial \beta_k} = X_{ik}.$$

This gives:

$$\frac{\partial^2 \ell_n(\beta)}{\partial \beta_j \partial \beta_k} = \sum_{i=1}^{n} X_{ij} \frac{\partial}{\partial \mu_i} \left[\frac{(Z_i - \mu_i)}{V(\mu_i)a(\phi)} \frac{\partial \mu_i}{\partial \eta_i} \right] \frac{\partial \mu_i}{\partial \eta_i} X_{ik}.$$

In the case of a canonical link function, we note that $\frac{\partial \mu_i}{\partial \eta_i} = V(\mu_i)$, and so:

$$\frac{\partial^2 \ell_n(\beta)}{\partial \beta_j \partial \beta_k} = \sum_{i=1}^{n} X_{ij} \frac{\partial}{\partial \mu_i} \left[\frac{(Z_i - \mu_i)}{a(\phi)} \right] V(\mu_i) X_{ik}$$

$$= -\frac{1}{a(\phi)} \sum_{i=1}^{n} X_{ij} V(\mu_i) X_{ik}.$$

Thus, we indeed recover the expression of $\partial^2 \ell_n(\beta)/\partial\beta\partial\beta^{\top}$ cited in equation [2.13], as expected.

The next section briefly revisits the binomial and Poisson regression models. These two models are arguably the most widely used examples of generalized linear regression models in applied contexts (excluding the special case of the Gaussian linear model). A wide range of books have been dedicated to studying them. Interested readers can, for example, refer to any one of [DOB 10, DEJ 08, HIL 09, HOS 00, MCC 89].

2.4. Binomial regression

2.4.1. *Logit link function*

In the case of the binomial regression model, the response variable Z_i follows a binomial distribution $\mathcal{B}(m_i, \pi_i)$. The parameter $\pi_i \in [0, 1]$ depends on the explanatory variables $\mathbf{X}_i$, and so we shall write $\pi_i = p(\mathbf{X}_i)$. The expected value of Z_i given $\mathbf{X}_i$

$$\mu_i = \mathbb{E}(Z_i | \mathbf{X}_i) = m_i p(\mathbf{X}_i)$$

is related to the linear predictor $\beta^{\top}\mathbf{X}_i$ via the link function g by setting: $g(\mu_i) = \beta^{\top}\mathbf{X}_i$. Hence, the binomial regression model is fully specified by:

$$\forall i = 1, \ldots, n, \quad \begin{cases} Z_i \sim \mathcal{B}(m_i, p(\mathbf{X}_i)) \\ g(\mu_i) = \beta^{\top}\mathbf{X}_i \end{cases}$$

We still need to choose g. The most widely used link function is the logistic function (we saw in Example 2.2 that this is in fact the canonical link function):

$$g(\mu_i) = \ln\left(\frac{\mu_i}{m_i - \mu_i}\right) = \ln\left(\frac{p(\mathbf{X}_i)}{1 - p(\mathbf{X}_i)}\right) = \text{logit}(p(\mathbf{X}_i)) = \beta^{\top}\mathbf{X}_i.$$

We can express $p(\mathbf{X}_i)$ as a function of $\mathbf{X}_i$ by inverting the logistic function:

$$p(\mathbf{X}_i) = \frac{e^{\beta^{\top}\mathbf{X}_i}}{1 + e^{\beta^{\top}\mathbf{X}_i}}.$$

Figure 2.5 shows the logistic function $x \mapsto \mathrm{logit}(x) = \ln(\frac{x}{1-x})$ (from $]0,1[$ to $\mathbb{R}$), as well as its inverse function $x \mapsto \frac{e^x}{1+e^x}$ (from $\mathbb{R}$ to $]0,1[$). Figure 2.6 shows the function $x \mapsto \frac{e^{\beta x}}{1+e^{\beta x}}$ for a few selected values of β. Figure 2.7 shows the function $x \mapsto \frac{e^{\alpha+x}}{1+e^{\alpha+x}}$ for a few selected values of α.

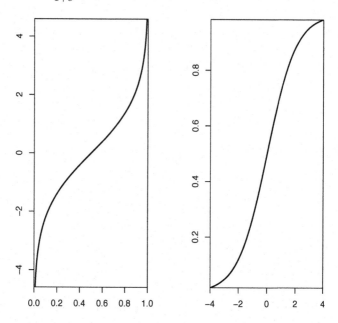

Figure 2.5. *Logit function (left) and its inverse function (right)*

REMARK.– Two other link functions are also used: the "probit" function, defined as the inverse of the standard Gaussian distribution function (which does not have an explicit expression), and the "log–log" function, defined by:

$$g(x) = \ln(-\ln(1-x)), \quad x \in]0,1[.$$

The logit, probit and log–log functions are shown in Figure 2.8. All three are fairly similar. The logistic function tends to be preferred, as it allows the coefficients β_j to be interpreted in terms of odds ratios.   □

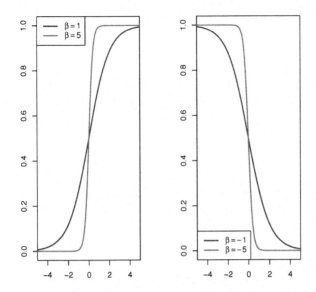

Figure 2.6. *Function* $x \mapsto \frac{e^{\beta x}}{1+e^{\beta x}}$ *with* $\beta = 1, 5$ *(left) and* $\beta = -1, -5$
(right). For a color version of the figure, please see
www.iste.co.uk/dupuy/countdata.zip

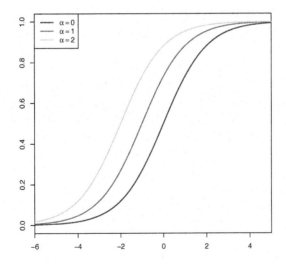

Figure 2.7. *Function* $x \mapsto \frac{e^{\alpha+x}}{1+e^{\alpha+x}}$ *with* $\alpha = 0, 1, 2$. *For a color version of*
the figure, please see www.iste.co.uk/dupuy/countdata.zip

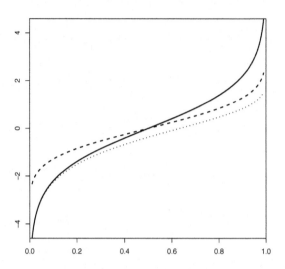

Figure 2.8. *Link functions: logit (solid), probit (dashes) and log–log (dots)*

2.4.2. *Estimation and statistical inference*

Suppose that we have n independent observations $(Z_1, \mathbf{X}_1), \ldots, (Z_n, \mathbf{X}_n)$ from the binomial regression model:

$$\forall i = 1, \ldots, n, \quad \begin{cases} Z_i \sim \mathcal{B}(m_i, p_\beta(\mathbf{X}_i)), \\ \operatorname{logit}(p_\beta(\mathbf{X}_i)) = \beta^\top \mathbf{X}_i \end{cases} \qquad [2.15]$$

We shall assume that $p < n$, as we did earlier for the linear regression. Let us first examine the identifiability of this model (we recall that a statistical model $(P_\theta, \theta \in \Theta)$ is said to be identifiable if the mapping $\theta \mapsto P_\theta$ is injective; intuitively, a model is identifiable whenever any two distinct parameters define distinct distributions).

THEOREM.– If $\mathbb{X}$ is full rank, then the model in equation [2.15] is identifiable.

PROOF.– Suppose that $p_\beta(\mathbf{X}_i) = p_{\tilde\beta}(\mathbf{X}_i)$ for all $i = 1, \ldots, n$. This implies that $\beta^\top \mathbf{X}_i = \tilde\beta^\top \mathbf{X}_i$ for all $i = 1, \ldots, n$, i.e. $\mathbb{X}\beta = \mathbb{X}\tilde\beta$, and so $\mathbb{X}(\beta - \tilde\beta) = 0$. If $\mathbb{X}$ is full rank, then its columns are a linearly independent set of vectors in $\mathbb{R}^n$, so $\beta = \tilde\beta$. Hence, the model is identifiable. $\square$

The parameter β is estimated by the maximum likelihood method. We calculated the likelihood of a binomial regression model earlier (section 2.3.1) from the probability density function of an arbitrary generalized linear model, but we shall repeat the calculation in the special case of the model in equation [2.15]. The likelihood is given by:

$$L_n(\beta) = \prod_{i=1}^{n} C_{m_i}^{Z_i} p_\beta(\mathbf{X}_i)^{Z_i} (1 - p_\beta(\mathbf{X}_i))^{m_i - Z_i},$$

which gives us the log-likelihood $\ell_n(\beta) = \ln L_n(\beta)$:

$$\ell_n(\beta) = \sum_{i=1}^{n} \left\{ Z_i \ln p_\beta(\mathbf{X}_i) + (m_i - Z_i) \ln(1 - p_\beta(\mathbf{X}_i)) + \ln C_{m_i}^{Z_i} \right\}$$

$$= \sum_{i=1}^{n} \left\{ Z_i \ln \left(\frac{p_\beta(\mathbf{X}_i)}{1 - p_\beta(\mathbf{X}_i)} \right) + m_i \ln(1 - p_\beta(\mathbf{X}_i)) + \ln C_{m_i}^{Z_i} \right\}$$

$$= \sum_{i=1}^{n} \left\{ Z_i \beta^\top \mathbf{X}_i - m_i \ln(1 + e^{\beta^\top \mathbf{X}_i}) + \ln C_{m_i}^{Z_i} \right\}.$$

The maximum likelihood estimator $\hat{\beta}_n$ of β is a solution of the equation:

$$\frac{\partial}{\partial \beta} \ell_n(\beta) \bigg|_{\beta = \hat{\beta}_n} = 0,$$

which can be rewritten as:

$$\sum_{i=1}^{n} X_{ij} \left(Z_i - m_i \frac{e^{\beta^\top \mathbf{X}_i}}{1 + e^{\beta^\top \mathbf{X}_i}} \right) = 0, \quad j = 1, \ldots, p,$$

or, alternatively:

$$\sum_{i=1}^{n} X_{ij}(Z_i - m_i p_\beta(\mathbf{X}_i)) = 0, \quad j = 1, \ldots, p.$$

This yields the formulas in equation [2.9], as expected.

2.5. Poisson regression

Suppose that we have n independent observations $(Z_1, \mathbf{X}_1), \ldots, (Z_n, \mathbf{X}_n)$ from the Poisson regression model:

$$\forall i = 1, \ldots, n, \quad \begin{cases} Z_i \sim \mathcal{P}(\lambda(\mathbf{X}_i)) \\ \ln \lambda(\mathbf{X}_i) = \beta^\top \mathbf{X}_i \end{cases}$$

This model is identifiable whenever the design matrix $\mathbb{X}$ is full rank. The likelihood is given by:

$$L_n(\beta) = \prod_{i=1}^{n} e^{-\lambda(\mathbf{X}_i)} \lambda(\mathbf{X}_i)^{Z_i} \frac{1}{Z_i!}.$$

The log-likelihood $\ell_n(\beta) = \ln L_n(\beta)$ is therefore:

$$\ell_n(\beta) = \sum_{i=1}^{n} \left\{ Z_i \beta^\top \mathbf{X}_i - e^{\beta^\top \mathbf{X}_i} - \ln(Z_i!) \right\}, \qquad [2.16]$$

and the score equations are:

$$\sum_{i=1}^{n} X_{ij}(Z_i - e^{\beta^\top \mathbf{X}_i}) = 0, \quad j = 1, \ldots, p.$$

Hence, we recover equation [2.10], as expected.

REMARK.– If the duration of observation varies from individual to individual, we may need to weigh the frequency of the observed events accordingly. Let E_i be the observation period (or "exposure") of the i-th individual. The model can be stated as follows:

$$\forall i = 1, \ldots, n, \quad \begin{cases} Z_i \sim \mathcal{P}(E_i \cdot \lambda(\mathbf{X}_i)) \\ \ln \lambda(\mathbf{X}_i) = \beta^\top \mathbf{X}_i \end{cases}$$

i.e. $Z_i \sim \mathcal{P}(\exp(\ln(E_i) + \beta^\top \mathbf{X}_i))$. The term $\ln(E_i)$ takes the form of an additional covariable with coefficient 1. $\qquad \square$

There are many other aspects of generalized linear models that deserve to be studied in their own right: model validation, methods for selecting variables and so on. Interested readers can refer to any of the following extremely comprehensive publications on these topics: [CAM 98, DOB 10, MCC 89]. The next section gives a few useful examples of R [RCO 17] functions that allow us to perform statistical inference from a generalized linear model.

2.6. Generalized linear models in R

In R, generalized linear models are implemented by the `glm` function. Below, we will illustrate how to use this function on the data set NMES1988 provided with the AER package [KLE 08]. As noted in section 1.5, we can access a description of these data by running the command:

```
help(NMES1988)
```

(a more complete description and a descriptive statistical analysis are given in [DEB 97]). These data were collected by a national survey on medical spending conducted in the United States from 1987 to 1988. The National Medical Expenditure Survey (NMES) considered 4,406 Medicare recipients aged 66 and over (Medicare is a health insurance system managed by the American federal government on behalf of over-65s).

For each survey participant, a series of variables were recorded to quantify their healthcare consumption. Specifically, the following numbers were recorded: office visits to a physician, office visits to a non-physician, outpatient appointments[2] with a physician, outpatient appointments with a non-physician, emergency care and hospital admissions. A set of explanatory variables were also observed for each individual. As an illustration, consider the following variables:

– gender (coded as 1 for women, 0 for men): `gender`,

– age (in years/10): `age`,

– marital status (coded as 1 if the patient is married, 0 otherwise): `fstatus`,

---

2 Outpatient appointments are defined as medical appointments performed at the hospital by hospital practitioners without involving hospitalization. This could for example represent an alternative to an office visit to a non-hospital practitioner, preparation for hospitalization, or post-hospitalization follow-up.

– duration of education (in years): school,

– income of the patient's household (in tens of thousands of US dollars): income,

– number of chronic diseases (cancer, diabetes, etc.) from which the patient suffers numchron,

– variable indicating whether the patient is covered by Medicaid (health insurance provided to low-income individuals and families), coded as 1 if the patient has Medicaid coverage, 0 if otherwise: med,

– variable indicating the patient's self-perception of their state of health (excellent, average, poor): health.

Suppose that we wish to establish a regression model for the count variable "physician office visits" (labeled as ofp below) as a function of these explanatory variables. We can visualize the distribution of ofp as a bar chart by running the following line of code:

```
plot(table(ofp),xlab="Number of physician office visits",
    ylab="Frequency")
```

which returns Figure 2.9.

We can construct an equivalent graphical representation with the following code:

```
visits.fac=factor(ofp,levels=0:max(ofp))
visits.tab=table(visits.fac)
barplot(visits.tab,xlab="Number of physician office
    visits",ylab="Frequency",col="lightblue")
```

which returns Figure 2.10.

The code after Figure 2.10 generates two representations of the number of office visits to a physician (response variable ofp) as a function of the number of chronic diseases (variable numchron). In the second representation, the transformation $\ln(\cdot + 1)$ is applied to the variable ofp (this performs a scale change that makes the graph easier to read).

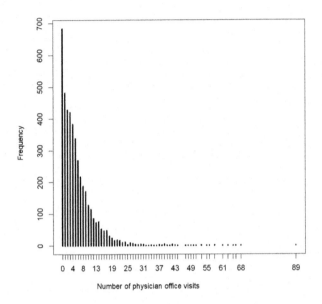

Figure 2.9. *Distribution of the frequency of the number of office visits to a physician (ofp)*

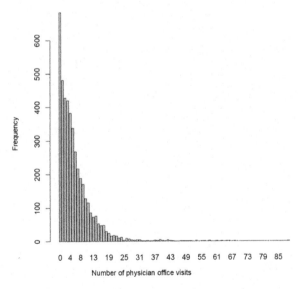

Figure 2.10. *Distribution of the frequency of the number of office visits to a physician (ofp)*

```
par(mfrow=c(1,2))
plot(ofp~numchron,xlab="Number of chronic diseases",ylab=
    "Physician office visits",main="numchron")
plot(log(ofp+1)~cutfac(numchron),xlab="Number of chronic
    diseases",ylab="Physician office visits (in log)",main
    ="numchron")
```

This code returns Figure 2.11.

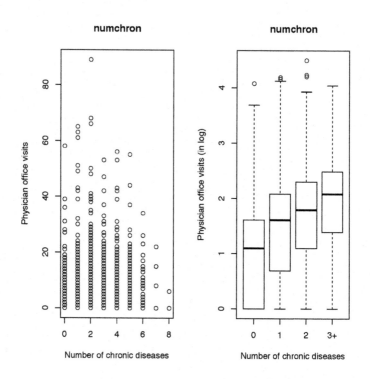

Figure 2.11. *Two representations of the number of office visits to a physician as a function of the number of chronic diseases*

Finally, the following code returns graphical representations of ofp as a function of multiple explanatory variables (Figure 2.12).

```
par(mfrow=c(2,2))
plot(log(ofp+1)~gender,varwidth=TRUE,xlab="Gender",ylab="
    Physician office visits (in log)",main="gender")
plot(log(ofp+1)~cutfac(numchron),xlab="Number of chronic
    diseases",ylab="Physician office visits (in log)",main
    ="numchron")
plot(log(ofp+1)~medicaid,varwidth=TRUE,xlab="Medicaid
    coverage",ylab="Physician office visits (in log)",main
    ="medicaid")
plot(log(ofp+1)~health,varwidth=TRUE,xlab="Self-perceived
    health status",ylab="Physician office visits (in log)
    ",main="health")
```

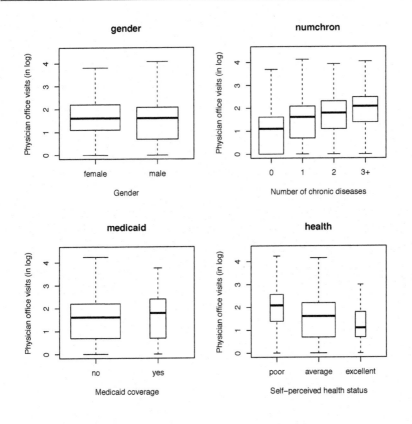

Figure 2.12. *Number of office visits to a physician as a function of multiple explanatory variables*

Suppose now that we wish to model the distribution of ofp as a function of the variables fstatus, school, income, numchron, med and health by performing a Poisson regression. We will recode the variable health in the form of two indicator variables: health1, which takes the value 1 if the self-perceived health status is poor and 0 if otherwise, and health2, which takes the value 1 if the self-perceived health status is excellent and 0 if otherwise. The model can now be stated as:

$$\begin{cases} Z_i \sim \mathcal{P}(\lambda(\mathbf{X}_i)) \\ \ln \lambda(\mathbf{X}_i) = \beta_1 + \beta_2\, \text{health1}_i + \beta_3\, \text{health2}_i + \beta_4\, \text{numchron}_i + \beta_5\, \text{age}_i \quad [2.17] \\ \qquad + \beta_6\, \text{gender}_i + \beta_7\, \text{fstatus}_i + \beta_8\, \text{school}_i + \beta_9\, \text{income}_i + \beta_{10}\, \text{med}_i \end{cases}$$

where health1_i, health2_i, numchron_i, etc., denote the values taken by the variables health1, health2, numchron, etc., on the i-th individual i, $i = 1, \ldots, 4406$.

In R, we can fit this model by running the following line of code, which is very similar to the code used earlier to fit a linear model using the lm function (section 1.5):

```
fit_pois=glm(ofp~health1+health2+numchron+age+gender+
    fstatus+school+income+med,family=poisson(link="log"))
```

We do not actually need to specify the link function, since the function ln is selected by default. The command family=poisson(link="log") can therefore be replaced by family=poisson. The code:

```
summary(fit_pois)
```

returns the output[3]:

---

3 Again, we do not attempt to interpret this output here. The objective of this section is simply to present a few useful functions for fitting generalized linear models in R.

```
Coefficients:
               Estimate Std. Error  z value  Pr(>|z|)
(Intercept)   1.3122787  0.0838913   15.643   < 2e-16  ***
health1       0.2924138  0.0175275   16.683   < 2e-16  ***
health2      -0.3816147  0.0303338  -12.581   < 2e-16  ***
numchron      0.1680809  0.0044698   37.604   < 2e-16  ***
age          -0.0394920  0.0103954   -3.799  0.000145  ***
gender        0.0849809  0.0141574    6.003  1.94e-09  ***
fstatus      -0.0201113  0.0145899   -1.378  0.168069
school        0.0349712  0.0018734   18.667   < 2e-16  ***
income        0.0002906  0.0022248    0.131  0.896074
med           0.1179474  0.0218939    5.387  7.15e-08  ***
---
Signif. codes:  0 '***' 0.001 '**' 0.01 '*' 0.05 '.' 0.1 '
     ' 1

(Dispersion parameter for poisson family taken to be 1)

    Null deviance: 26943  on 4405  degrees of freedom
Residual deviance: 23933  on 4396  degrees of freedom
AIC: 36729

Number of Fisher Scoring iterations: 5
```

2.6.1. Output of the glm function

First, we observe that the Fisher scoring algorithm converged to an approximation of $\hat{\beta}_n$ in five iterations. The output includes a reminder that the dispersion parameter ϕ is equal to 1 for the Poisson model.

We recall that the maximum likelihood estimator $\hat{\beta}_n$ is asymptotically distributed as a Gaussian vector $\mathcal{N}(\beta, \mathcal{I}_n(\hat{\beta}_n)^{-1})$, where:

$$\mathcal{I}_n(\hat{\beta}_n)^{-1} = \left(-\frac{\partial^2 \ell_n(\hat{\beta}_n)}{\partial \beta \partial \beta^\top} \right)^{-1}$$

$$= (\mathbb{X}^\top W(\hat{\beta}_n)\mathbb{X})^{-1}.$$

The term ℓ_n is given by equation [2.16] and $W(\beta)$ is the diagonal matrix with i-th diagonal term $\exp(\beta^\top \mathbf{X}_i)$, $i = 1, \ldots, n$ (with $n = 4,406$). The estimates of $\beta_1, \ldots, \beta_{10}$ are listed in the "Estimate" column. The "Std. error" column (short for "standard error") gives estimates of the (asymptotic) standard deviations of the $\hat{\beta}_{n,i}$ (i.e. the square root of the diagonal terms of $\mathcal{I}_n(\hat{\beta}_n)^{-1}$).

REMARK.– The log-likelihood $\ell_n(\hat{\beta}_n)$ of the estimated model is returned by the logLik function:

```
logLik(fit_pois)
'log Lik.' -18354.36 (df=10)
```

The matrix $\mathcal{I}_n(\hat{\beta}_n)^{-1}$ is returned by vcov(fit_pois). $\square$

The "z value" column lists the values of the Wald statistic, which tests $H_0 : \beta_i = 0$ against $H_1 : \beta_i \neq 0$. Under H_0, z is asymptotically distributed like $\mathcal{N}(0, 1)$. For a test with an asymptotic significance level of α, we therefore need to compare $|z|$ with the quantile of order $1 - \alpha/2$ of $\mathcal{N}(0, 1)$. The corresponding p-values are listed in the column "Pr($> |z|$)". We reject H_0 whenever the p-value is less than α.

The output also includes two deviance values. The null deviance is defined as the deviance of the model:

$$\forall i = 1, \ldots, n, \quad \begin{cases} Z_i \sim \mathcal{P}(\lambda(\mathbf{X}_i)) \\ \ln \lambda(\mathbf{X}_i) = \beta_1 \end{cases}$$

The linear predictor in this model is simply the constant variable. The number of degrees of freedom is defined as the difference between the sample size n and the number p of model parameters. Here, $p = 1$, which gives a number of degrees of freedom equal to $4,406 - 1 = 4,405$. The residual deviance is the deviance of the model in equation [2.17], which has $4,406 - 10 = 4,396$ degrees of freedom. From these results, we can construct a deviance test of:

$$H_0 : \beta_2 = \ldots = \beta_{10} = 0$$

against

$$H_1 : \text{ there exists } i \in \{2, \ldots, 10\} \text{ such that } \beta_i \neq 0.$$

The test statistic is equal to $26,943 - 23,933 = 3,010$. This statistic is compared to the quantile of order $1 - \alpha$ of a χ^2 distribution with nine degrees of freedom. The required quantile is returned by the qchisq function. For a test with an asymptotic significance level of 0.05, it has the value:

```
qchisq(0.95,9)
[1] 16.91898
```

Hence, the null hypothesis H_0 is rejected. The same test can also be performed using the anova function after fitting the model under H_0. The code:

```
fit_poisH0=glm(ofp~1,family=poisson)
anova(fit_poisH0,fit_pois,test="Chisq")
```

returns the test statistic and the corresponding p-value:

```
Analysis of Deviance Table

Model 1: ofp ~ 1
Model 2: ofp ~ health1 + health2 + numchron + age +
    gender + fstatus + school + income + med
  Resid. Df Resid. Dev Df Deviance  Pr(>Chi)
1      4405      26943
2      4396      23933  9   3009.6 < 2.2e-16 ***
---
Signif. codes: 0 '***' 0.001 '**' 0.01 '*' 0.05 '.' 0.1 '
    ' 1
```

2.6.2. *Tests between nested models*

More generally, the anova function allows us to compare any two nested models by performing a deviance test. Suppose that we wish to test the non-significance of the health variable for the model in equation [2.17]:

$$H_0 : \beta_2 = \beta_3 = 0 \text{ against } H_1 : \beta_2 \neq 0 \text{ or } \beta_3 \neq 0.$$

The code:

```
fit_poisH0=update(fit_pois,formula=.~.-health1-health2)
anova(fit_poisH0,fit_pois,test="Chisq")
```

estimates the model under H_0 and then computes the deviance statistic (under H_0, this statistic asymptotically follows a χ^2_2 distribution). The anova function returns the output:

```
Analysis of Deviance Table

Model 1: ofp ~ numchron + age + gender + fstatus + school
    + income + med
Model 2: ofp ~ health1 + health2 + numchron + age +
    gender + fstatus + school + income + med
  Resid. Df Resid. Dev Df Deviance  Pr(>Chi)
1      4398      24397
2      4396      23933  2   463.61 < 2.2e-16 ***
---
Signif.codes: 0'***' 0.001'**' 0.01'*' 0.05 '.' 0.1 '' 1
```

Alternatively, we could use the lrtest function from the lmtest package [ZEI 02], which performs a likelihood-ratio test (which is equivalent to the deviance test). The syntax of this command is as follows:

```
lrtest(fit_poisH0,fit_pois)
```

We of course obtain the same result as before, although the results are presented slightly differently:

```
Likelihood ratio test

Model 1: ofp ~ numchron + age + gender + fstatus + school
    + income + med
Model 2: ofp ~ health1 + health2 + numchron + age +
    gender + fstatus + school + income + med
  #Df LogLik Df  Chisq Pr(>Chisq)
1   8 -18586
2  10 -18354  2 463.61  < 2.2e-16 ***
---
Signif.codes: 0 '***' 0.001'**' 0.01 '*' 0.05'.' 0.1 '' 1
```

Finally, we can use a Wald test to compare nested models (the `waldtest` function from the `lmtest` package). The following R code:

```
waldtest(fit_poisH0,formula=.~.+health1+health2,test="
    Chisq")
```

returns the output:

```
Wald test

Model 1: ofp ~ numchron + age + gender + fstatus + school
    + income + med
Model 2: ofp ~ numchron + age + gender + fstatus + school
    + income + med + health1 + health2

  Res.Df Df  Chisq Pr(>Chisq)
1   4398
2   4396  2 455.21  < 2.2e-16 ***
---
Signif.codes: 0'***' 0.001'**' 0.01'*' 0.05'.' 0.1 '' 1
```

2.6.3. Automatic variable selection

We note that the `glm` function computes the Akaike information criterion (AIC). This criterion can be applied to perform automatic variable selection using the `stepAIC` function from the `MASS` package [VEN 02]:

```
stepAIC(fit_pois)
```

The output of this command lists each of the steps taken until a model is obtained for which the AIC cannot be reduced any further by adding or removing explanatory variables:

```
Start:   AIC=36728.73
ofp ~ health1 + health2 + numchron + age + gender +
    fstatus + school + income + med

            Df Deviance    AIC
- income     1    23933  36727
- fstatus    1    23935  36729
```

```
<none>                23933 36729
- age          1      23948 36741
- med          1      23962 36755
- gender       1      23970 36763
- health2      1      24110 36903
- health1      1      24201 36994
- school       1      24287 37081
- numchron     1      25266 38059


Step:   AIC=36726.74
ofp ~ health1 + health2 + numchron + age + gender +
    fstatus + school + med


              Df Deviance   AIC
- fstatus      1     23935 36727
<none>               23933 36727
- age          1     23948 36739
- med          1     23962 36753
- gender       1     23970 36761
- health2      1     24110 36902
- health1      1     24201 36992
- school       1     24304 37095
- numchron     1     25266 38057


Step:   AIC=36726.64
ofp ~ health1 + health2 + numchron + age + gender +
    school + med


              Df Deviance   AIC
<none>               23935 36727
- age          1     23948 36737
- med          1     23966 36755
- gender       1     23985 36775
- health2      1     24112 36901
- health1      1     24202 36992
- school       1     24304 37093
- numchron     1     25269 38058


Call:   glm(formula=ofp~health1+health2+numchron+age+
    gender+school+med,family=poisson(link="log"))


Coefficients:
(Intercept) health1 health2  numchron age       gender
    school
1.27381      0.29210 -0.38094 0.16815 -0.03614  0.09234
    0.03483
med
```

```
0.12174

Degrees of Freedom: 4405 Total (i.e. Null);   4398
    Residual
Null Deviance:      26940
Residual Deviance: 23940        AIC: 36730
```

3

Overdispersion in Count Data

3.1. Introduction

The mean of a Poisson distribution is equal to its variance – we say that this distribution is equidispersed. Given a Poisson regression model $Z \sim \mathcal{P}(\lambda(\mathbf{X}))$, where $\mathbf{X}$ denotes a set of explanatory variables, the equidispersion property can be represented by the equation:

$$\mathbb{E}(Z|\mathbf{X}) = \text{var}(Z|\mathbf{X}),$$

which states that the conditional expected value and variance of Z are equal given $\mathbf{X}$.

Returning to the NMES1988 data from the US national survey on medical expenditure [DEB 97], we consider the ofp variable (the number of office visits to a physician). Figure 3.1 shows the frequency distribution of ofp. One very empirical way of checking whether the conditional distribution of ofp given $\mathbf{X}$ is equidispersed is to estimate the mean $\mathbb{E}(Z|\mathbf{X} = \mathbf{x})$ and the variance $\text{var}(Z|\mathbf{X} = \mathbf{x})$ for each $\mathbf{X} = \mathbf{x}$ by the empirical mean and variance of the observations Z_i of ofp such that $\{\mathbf{X}_i = \mathbf{x}\}$ and then plot the pairs (estimated mean, estimated variance) in the plane. If the equidispersion property is satisfied, then the scatterplot should have approximately the same form as the line $y = x$.

To restrict the data to finitely many values of $\mathbf{x}$, any quantitative explanatory variables (e.g. age and income) or integer-valued explanatory variables (e.g.

school and numchron) are discretized into a small set of categories. This gives a new set of qualitative explanatory variables, whose values are crossed to give N distinct categories $\mathbf{x}_1, \ldots, \mathbf{x}_N$.

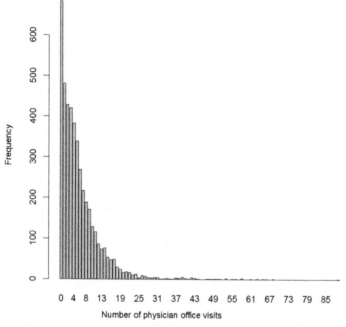

Poisson-ofp2

Figure 3.1. *Frequency distribution of the number of office visits to a physician (ofp)*

This procedure is applied to the variables health, med, age and numchron (many of the categories $\mathbf{x}_j$ would only contain 0 or 1 individuals if we crossed more variables, which is why we restrict ourselves to this small set; however, if necessary, we can repeat the procedure on other subsets of the explanatory variables). Thus, we need to find the empirical mean and variance of the observations of ofp for every category $\mathbf{x}$ obtained by crossing health, med, age and numchron and then plot the corresponding pairs (empirical mean, empirical variance) in the plane. The result is shown in Figure 3.2.

The blue line $y = x$ in this figure shows the case of perfect equidispersion, $\mathrm{var}(Z|\mathbf{X}) = \mathbb{E}(Z|\mathbf{X})$. The red line is the least squares line obtained by performing a simple linear regression of the empirical variance on the empirical mean.

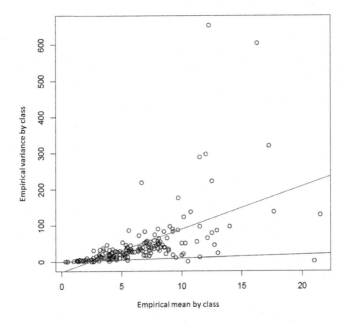

Figure 3.2. *Empirical mean and variance within each class* x *obtained after segmentation of the variables* health, med, age *and* numchron. *For a color version of the figure, please see www.iste.co.uk/dupuy/countdata.zip*

This graph shows that, for almost every value of x, the empirical variance of the Z_i in the class x is higher than their empirical mean (the points mostly lie above the line $y = x$). Hence, the data are overdispersed.

Overdispersion can arise due to various reasons. In this book, we consider two of the most important sources of overdispersed data, namely: i) the presence of unobserved heterogeneity in the data and ii) zero inflation (which is the focus of Chapter 4).

Unobserved heterogeneity can take many forms. For example, let us consider the model:

$$Z_i \sim \begin{cases} \mathcal{P}(\lambda_0) \text{ if } X_i = 0 \\ \mathcal{P}(\lambda_1) \text{ if } X_i = 1 \end{cases}$$

where X_i follows a Bernoulli distribution with parameter π_i and $\lambda_0 \neq \lambda_1$ (the same reasoning would apply if λ_0 and λ_1 depend on the individual i, for instance, via the explanatory variables; any such dependence is omitted here to simplify the notation). The quantity X_i is a factor of the heterogeneity of the observations Z_i. Indeed, the distribution of the Z_i changes according to whether $X_i = 0$ or $X_i = 1$ as follows: $Z_i | X_i = 0 \sim \mathcal{P}(\lambda_0)$ and $Z_i | X_i = 1 \sim \mathcal{P}(\lambda_1)$.

Suppose now that X_i is unobserved and that we only know the value of Z_i or that X_i is observed but its effect is not modeled. Then:

$$\begin{aligned} \mathbb{E}(Z_i) &= \mathbb{E}[\mathbb{E}[Z_i | X_i]] \\ &= \mathbb{E}(\lambda_0(1 - X_i) + \lambda_1 X_i) \\ &= \pi_i \lambda_1 + (1 - \pi_i)\lambda_0 \end{aligned}$$

and

$$\begin{aligned} \mathrm{var}(Z_i) &= \mathbb{E}[\mathrm{var}(Z_i | X_i)] + \mathrm{var}(\mathbb{E}[Z_i | X_i]) \\ &= \mathbb{E}(Z_i) + \mathrm{var}(\lambda_0 + (\lambda_1 - \lambda_0)X_i) \\ &= \mathbb{E}(Z_i) + (\lambda_1 - \lambda_0)^2 \pi_i(1 - \pi_i). \end{aligned}$$

If $\pi_i \neq 0, 1$ (in other words, if X_i effectively induces some heterogeneity in the distribution of Z_i), then:

$$\mathrm{var}(Z_i) > \mathbb{E}(Z_i),$$

and the marginal distribution of Z_i is overdispersed (whereas the conditional distributions of $Z_i | X_i = 0$ and $Z_i | X_i = 1$ are equidispersed). If X_i is unobserved or neglected and the heterogeneity that it induces in the distribution of the observations is not taken into account, then any variability in Z_i explained by X_i is not captured by the model. This unexplained variability is ultimately reflected in the overdispersion.

Unobserved heterogeneity can also arise from the omission of one or several key explanatory variables (or interactions between explanatory variables) from the linear predictor of the model. We can perform a numerical mini-experiment as an illustration.

Suppose that we simulate $n = 5,000$ independent realizations of the variables $X_1 \sim \mathcal{U}[0, 1]$ (where $\mathcal{U}[0, 1]$ denotes the uniform distribution on the interval $[0, 1]$), $X_2 \sim \mathcal{U}[0, 1]$ and $X_3 \sim \mathcal{N}(0, 1)$. We then simulate n independent counts $Z_i \sim \mathcal{P}(\lambda(\mathbf{X}_i))$, where $\mathbf{X}_i = (X_{i1}, X_{i2}, X_{i3})$ and $\lambda(\mathbf{X}_i) = \exp(\beta_0 + \beta_1 X_{i1} + \beta_2 X_{i2} + \beta_3 X_{i3})$.

Next, we estimate $\mathbb{E}(Z|\mathbf{X} = \mathbf{x})$ and $\text{var}(Z|\mathbf{X} = \mathbf{x})$ using the procedure described above. To do this, each of the variables X_1, X_2, X_3 is discretized into eight categories. This gives $N = 8^3 = 512$ classes, $\mathbf{x}_1, \ldots, \mathbf{x}_N$, allowing us to calculate an empirical estimate of $\mathbb{E}(Z|\mathbf{X} = \mathbf{x}_j)$ and $\text{var}(Z|\mathbf{X} = \mathbf{x}_j)$, $j = 1, \ldots, N$. The scatterplot of the N estimated pairs $(\mathbb{E}(Z|\mathbf{X} = \mathbf{x}_j), \text{var}(Z|\mathbf{X} = \mathbf{x}_j))$ is shown by blue circles in Figure 3.3. The least squares line obtained by regressing the empirical variances on the empirical means is shown as a dashed line; this line estimates the relation between the conditional mean and the conditional variance of the distribution of Z_i given (X_1, X_2, X_3). The solid line $y = x$ shows the equidispersed case.

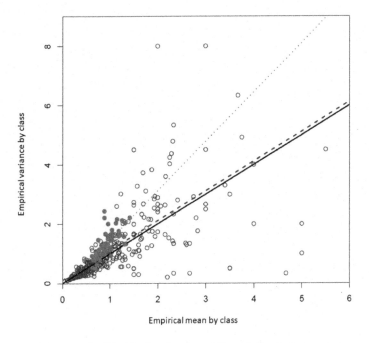

Figure 3.3. *Empirical estimates of the relation between* $\mathbb{E}(Z|\mathbf{X} = \mathbf{x})$ *and var*$(Z|\mathbf{X} = \mathbf{x})$. *For a color version of the figure, please see www.iste.co.uk/dupuy/countdata.zip*

Now, let us re-estimate the conditional mean and variance of Z while omitting X_3 (the classes $\mathbf{x}_j$ are constructed by crossing the categories of the discretized versions of X_1 and X_2). The cloud of estimated points $(\mathbb{E}(Z|\mathbf{X} = \mathbf{x}_j), \text{var}(Z|\mathbf{X} = \mathbf{x}_j))$ is shown as red dots in Figure 3.3. The corresponding least-squares line is plotted as a dotted line.

This illustrates that omitting an explanatory variable in the linear predictor $\lambda(\mathbf{X}_i)$ leads to overdispersion in the observations of Z (in other words, the variance is greater than the mean). By contrast, when every explanatory variable is included in the predictor, we recover the equidispersion property of Z.

REMARK.– As we noted above, overdispersion can arise due to various reasons (omission of explanatory variables or interactions, presence of outliers, model misspecification, etc.). Readers interested in exploring this topic further can refer to [HIL 11]. □

Why is overdispersion a problem? To answer this question, we note that if we fit a Poisson model to overdispersed data, then we will underestimate the variance of the estimators of the β_j and hence underestimate the "standard errors" that appear in the denominator of the Wald test, as well as the confidence interval formulas. One possible ramification is that non-significant explanatory variables may appear to be significant.

The next part of this chapter presents two models that are widely used for overdispered count data.

3.2. The quasi-Poisson model

3.2.1. *Definition*

We consider again the Poisson regression model:

$$\forall i = 1, \ldots, n, \quad \begin{cases} Z_i \sim \mathcal{P}(\lambda(\mathbf{X}_i)) \\ \ln \lambda(\mathbf{X}_i) = \beta^\top \mathbf{X}_i \end{cases}$$

The maximum likelihood estimator $\hat{\beta}_n$ satisfies the score equation:

$$\sum_{i=1}^{n} \mathbf{X}_i(Z_i - e^{\beta^\top \mathbf{X}_i}) = 0,$$

which is obtained by differentiating the log-likelihood of the model. We know that $\hat{\beta}_n$ is a consistent estimator of β. In fact, $\hat{\beta}_n$ is consistent even when the distribution of $Z_i|\mathbf{X}_i$ is not Poisson, provided that the conditional expectation of Z_i is of the form $\mathbb{E}(Z_i|\mathbf{X}_i) = e^{\beta^\top \mathbf{X}_i}$. For $\hat{\beta}_n$ to be consistent, it suffices for $\mathbb{E}(\mathbf{X}_i(Z_i - e^{\beta^\top \mathbf{X}_i})) = 0$, which is the case whenever $\mathbb{E}(Z_i|\mathbf{X}_i) = e^{\beta^\top \mathbf{X}_i}$.

REMARK.– The fact that $\hat{\beta}_n$ is consistent whenever $\mathbb{E}(\mathbf{X}_i(Z_i - e^{\beta^\top \mathbf{X}_i})) = 0$ can be shown using an argument from asymptotic statistics, described briefly below (interested readers can find more details in [VAN 98]). Let:

$$S_n(\beta) = \frac{1}{n} \sum_{i=1}^{n} \mathbf{X}_i(Z_i - e^{\beta^\top \mathbf{X}_i}),$$

and $S(\beta) = \mathbb{E}(\mathbf{X}_i(Z_i - e^{\beta^\top \mathbf{X}_i}))$.

By the law of large numbers, $S_n(\beta)$ converges in probability to $S(\beta)$. If this convergence is sufficiently "strong" (e.g. uniform convergence in β; see [VAN 98]), and if the model is identifiable, then the solution $\hat{\beta}_n$ of $S_n(\hat{\beta}_n) = 0$ converges in probability to the unique solution of $S(\beta) = 0$.

To gain some intuition, we write β_0 for the true value of the parameter. If the conditional expectation of Z_i is of the form $\mathbb{E}(Z_i|\mathbf{X}_i) = e^{\beta_0^\top \mathbf{X}_i}$, then:

$$\begin{aligned}
S(\beta_0) &= \mathbb{E}(\mathbf{X}_i(Z_i - e^{\beta_0^\top \mathbf{X}_i})) \\
&= \mathbb{E}[\mathbb{E}(\mathbf{X}_i(Z_i - e^{\beta_0^\top \mathbf{X}_i})|\mathbf{X}_i)] \\
&= \mathbb{E}[\mathbf{X}_i\{\mathbb{E}(Z_i|\mathbf{X}_i) - e^{\beta_0^\top \mathbf{X}_i}\}] \\
&= 0,
\end{aligned}$$

and $\hat{\beta}_n$ converges in probability to β_0. □

This robustness of $\hat{\beta}_n$ with respect to the distribution of Z_i implies that we can estimate β by $\hat{\beta}_n$ even when the true distribution of Z_i is not a Poisson distribution, provided that $\mathbb{E}(Z_i|\mathbf{X}_i) = e^{\beta^\top \mathbf{X}_i}$. This observation motivates the quasi-Poisson model described below.

Suppose that we have a count variable Z_i such that $Z_i|\mathbf{X}_i$ has the distribution G_i. We do not assume anything specific about the distribution G_i (in particular, we do not assume that G_i is a Poisson distribution). We only assume that the expected value of Z_i given $\mathbf{X}_i$ is of the form:

$$\mathbb{E}(Z_i|\mathbf{X}_i) = e^{\beta^\top \mathbf{X}_i}.$$

Let $\omega_i = \mathrm{var}(Z_i|\mathbf{X}_i)$ (without assuming equidispersion). The quasi-Poisson model is defined in terms of the first two moments of G_i as follows:

$$\forall i = 1, \ldots, n, \quad \begin{cases} Z_i|\mathbf{X}_i \sim G_i \\ \mathbb{E}(Z_i|\mathbf{X}_i) = e^{\beta^\top \mathbf{X}_i} \\ \mathrm{var}(Z_i|\mathbf{X}_i) = \omega_i \end{cases} \qquad [3.1]$$

3.2.2. Quasi-maximum likelihood

In the quasi-Poisson model, we can estimate β by the solution of the equation:

$$\sum_{i=1}^{n} \mathbf{X}_i(Z_i - e^{\beta^\top \mathbf{X}_i}) = 0.$$

The estimator thus obtained, denoted as $\hat{\beta}_n^Q$, is called the quasi-maximum likelihood estimator [WED 74], since $\hat{\beta}_n^Q$ follows from the likelihood equation of a Poisson model even when G_i is left unspecified.

REMARK.– Clearly, $\hat{\beta}_n^Q$ is equal to the maximum likelihood estimator in any Poisson model, since the estimation equations are the same. However, the estimated variance is not the same, as shown below.   □

Suppose that $\mu_i = \mathbb{E}(Z_i|\mathbf{X}_i)$ is indeed given by $e^{\beta^\top \mathbf{X}_i}$. Then, asymptotically, $\hat{\beta}_n^Q$ is approximately distributed like the Gaussian vector

$\mathcal{N}(\beta, \text{var}(\hat{\beta}_n^Q))$ (see [CAM 98]), where:

$$\text{var}(\hat{\beta}_n^Q) = \left(\sum_{i=1}^{n} \mu_i \mathbf{X}_i \mathbf{X}_i^\top\right)^{-1} \left(\sum_{i=1}^{n} \omega_i \mathbf{X}_i \mathbf{X}_i^\top\right) \left(\sum_{i=1}^{n} \mu_i \mathbf{X}_i \mathbf{X}_i^\top\right)^{-1} \quad [3.2]$$

REMARK.– In cases with equidispersion (in particular, whenever $Z_i | \mathbf{X}_i \sim \mathcal{P}(\mu_i)$), we have $\omega_i = \mu_i$, and $\text{var}(\hat{\beta}_n^Q)$ becomes:

$$\text{var}(\hat{\beta}_n^Q) = \left(\sum_{i=1}^{n} \mu_i \mathbf{X}_i \mathbf{X}_i^\top\right)^{-1}.$$

This recovers the variance–covariance matrix of the maximum likelihood estimator $\hat{\beta}_n$ in a Poisson model. Thus, even if the distribution $Z_i | \mathbf{X}_i$ is not a Poisson distribution, we can make inferences about β based on $\hat{\beta}_n$ and its asymptotic properties in the Poisson model, provided that the condition $\omega_i = \mu_i = e^{\beta^\top \mathbf{X}_i}$ holds. □

To make inferences regarding β in the quasi-Poisson model, we need to be able to estimate the variance in equation [3.2], which depends on the unknowns $\mu_i = \mathbb{E}(Z_i | \mathbf{X}_i)$ and $\omega_i = \text{var}(Z_i | \mathbf{X}_i) = \mathbb{E}[(Z_i - \mu_i)^2 | \mathbf{X}_i]$.

We can estimate μ_i by $\hat{\mu}_i = e^{\hat{\beta}_n^{Q\top} \mathbf{X}_i}$. If we want to avoid making any assumptions about the form of $\omega_i = \text{var}(Z_i | \mathbf{X}_i)$, then we can estimate ω_i by $(Z_i - \hat{\mu}_i)^2$ and equation [3.2] by:

$$\widehat{\text{var}(\hat{\beta}_n^Q)} = \left(\sum_{i=1}^{n} \hat{\mu}_i \mathbf{X}_i \mathbf{X}_i^\top\right)^{-1} \left(\sum_{i=1}^{n} (Z_i - \hat{\mu}_i)^2 \mathbf{X}_i \mathbf{X}_i^\top\right) \left(\sum_{i=1}^{n} \hat{\mu}_i \mathbf{X}_i \mathbf{X}_i^\top\right)^{-1}.$$

REMARK.– This estimator is sometimes called the sandwich estimator, since it is of the form $\mathbf{A}^{-1}\mathbf{B}\mathbf{A}^{-1}$; the matrix $\mathbf{B}$ is "sandwiched" between $\mathbf{A}^{-1}$ and $\mathbf{A}^{-1}$. Some authors also call it the robust estimator.

To estimate $\text{var}(\hat{\beta}_n^Q)$ without making any assumptions about ω_i, we can also use the bootstrap method (interested readers can find more information in [CAM 98]). □

Another approach widely used in practice is to assume that ω_i is of the specific form:

$$\omega_i = \text{var}(Z_i|\mathbf{X}_i) = \phi\mathbb{E}(Z_i|\mathbf{X}_i) = \phi\mu_i, \qquad [3.3]$$

where ϕ is a dispersion parameter. Overdispersion corresponds to the case where $\phi > 1$. If $\phi < 1$, we instead speak of underdispersion. The advantage of this approach is that it provides a numerical value that quantifies the overdispersion. Under the hypothesis in equation [3.3], $\text{var}(\hat{\beta}_n^Q)$ becomes:

$$\text{var}(\hat{\beta}_n^Q) = \phi\left(\sum_{i=1}^{n}\mu_i\mathbf{X}_i\mathbf{X}_i^\top\right)^{-1}.$$

We note that the variance of $\hat{\beta}_n^Q$ is increased by a factor of ϕ relative to the variance of $\hat{\beta}_n$ in the Poisson model. Therefore, an explanatory variable that is significant in an overdispersed Poisson model (the case where $\phi > 1$) is not necessarily significant after performing a more suitable fitting with a quasi-Poisson model.

In general, ϕ is unknown. Since we have that:

$$\phi = \frac{\text{var}(Z_i|\mathbf{X}_i)}{\mathbb{E}(Z_i|\mathbf{X}_i)} = \mathbb{E}\left[\frac{(Z_i - \mu_i)^2}{\mu_i}|\mathbf{X}_i\right],$$

a natural way of estimating ϕ is given by:

$$\widehat{\phi} = \frac{1}{n-p}\sum_{i=1}^{n}\frac{(Z_i - \hat{\mu}_i)^2}{\hat{\mu}_i}, \qquad [3.4]$$

and we can estimate $\text{var}(\hat{\beta}_n^Q)$ by:

$$\widehat{\text{var}(\hat{\beta}_n^Q)} = \hat{\phi}\left(\sum_{i=1}^{n}\hat{\mu}_i\mathbf{X}_i\mathbf{X}_i^\top\right)^{-1}.$$

REMARK.– Fitting a quasi-Poisson model is ultimately equivalent to fitting a Poisson model and then correcting the variance and standard error terms by ϕ and $\sqrt{\phi}$, respectively.

In R, the quasi-Poisson model is implemented by calling the glm function with the option "family=quasipoisson()."   □

It is possible to define a likelihood for the quasi-Poisson model, but this is not particularly useful in practice. Consider the probability density function:

$$f(z_i; \beta, \phi) = \exp\left(\frac{z_i \beta^\top \mathbf{X}_i - e^{\beta^\top \mathbf{X}_i}}{\phi} + c(z_i, \phi)\right), \quad i = 1, \ldots, n. \quad [3.5]$$

Then, $\mu_i = \mathbb{E}(Z_i | \mathbf{X}_i) = e^{\beta^\top \mathbf{X}_i}$ and $\omega_i = \mathrm{var}(Z_i | \mathbf{X}_i) = \phi \mu_i$. The model in equation [3.5] therefore coincides with the quasi-Poisson model in equation [3.1], where ω_i is as in equation [3.3]. It is straightforward to check that the maximum likelihood estimator $\tilde{\beta}_n$ of the model resulting from equation [3.5] satisfies:

$$\frac{1}{\phi} \sum_{i=1}^n \mathbf{X}_i (Z_i - e^{\beta^\top \mathbf{X}_i}) = 0.$$

Up to the multiplicative constant $1/\phi$, this is the same as the estimation equation of the quasi-Poisson model. Hence, $\tilde{\beta}_n$ and $\hat{\beta}_n^Q$ coincide. Furthermore, both are approximately distributed like $\mathcal{N}(0, \phi \left(\sum_{i=1}^n \mu_i \mathbf{X}_i \mathbf{X}_i^\top\right)^{-1})$.

Since we can define a density function for the quasi-Poisson model, it might occur to us to try to estimate ϕ by maximizing the likelihood. To do this, we would need to know $c(z_i, \phi)$. However, the constraint

$$\sum_{z_i=0}^\infty f(z_i; \beta, \phi) = \sum_{z_i=0}^\infty \exp\left(\frac{z_i \beta^\top \mathbf{X}_i - e^{\beta^\top \mathbf{X}_i}}{\phi} + c(z_i, \phi)\right) = 1$$

does not give us an explicit expression for $c(z_i, \phi)$. Instead, we must return to the estimator in equation [3.4], whose construction only requires the assumption $\omega_i = \phi \mu_i$ on the first two moments of the distribution of Z_i. Thus, defining a density function for the quasi-Poisson model is ultimately not helpful for making inferences about β.

Another approach to accounting for overdispersion in a Poisson model is to view its parameter as a random variable with its own probability distribution.

The underlying idea of this approach is that introducing an additional source of variability into the model allows us to provide a better explanation of any excess dispersion in the observations.

3.3. The negative binomial regression model

Let U_i be a random variable with a gamma distribution $G(1, \nu)$ (see equation [2.3] for the density function of U_i). Suppose that Z_i given U_i follows a Poisson distribution with parameter $\mu_i U_i$, where $\mu_i > 0$ is fixed. Notationally, we write:

$$Z_i | U_i \sim \mathcal{P}(\mu_i U_i).$$

We observe that $\mathbb{E}(Z_i) = \mathbb{E}[\mathbb{E}[Z_i | U_i]] = \mathbb{E}[\mu_i U_i] = \mu_i \mathbb{E}[U_i] = \mu_i$. In practice, the variable U_i is unobserved. It allows us to introduce heterogeneity between individuals by adding variability to the mean value of their response. Let us find the distribution of Z_i. For all $z \in \mathbb{N}$:

$$
\begin{aligned}
\mathbb{P}(Z_i = z) &= \int_0^\infty e^{-\mu_i u} \frac{(\mu_i u)^z}{z!} \frac{\nu^\nu}{\Gamma(\nu)} u^{\nu-1} e^{-u\nu} \, du \\
&= \frac{\nu^\nu \mu_i^z}{\Gamma(\nu) z!} \int_0^\infty e^{-(\mu_i + \nu)u} u^{z+\nu-1} \, du \\
&= \frac{\nu^\nu \mu_i^z}{\Gamma(\nu) z!} \frac{\Gamma(z+\nu)}{(\mu_i + \nu)^{z+\nu}} \\
&= \frac{\Gamma(z+\nu)}{\Gamma(\nu) z!} \left(\frac{\mu_i}{\nu + \mu_i} \right)^z \left(\frac{\nu}{\nu + \mu_i} \right)^\nu.
\end{aligned}
$$

Up to re-parameterization (e.g. by setting $\kappa = 1/\nu$ and $\mu = \mu_i$), this is the density function of the negative binomial distribution (equation [2.4]). The mean and the variance of Z_i are, respectively, given by:

$$\mathbb{E}(Z_i) = \mu_i$$

and

$$\text{var}(Z_i) = \mu_i(1 + \kappa \mu_i) = \mu_i + \kappa \mu_i^2. \tag{3.6}$$

We note that $\text{var}(Z_i) > \mathbb{E}(Z_i)$ (since $\kappa > 0$), which makes the negative binomial distribution an obvious choice for modeling overdispersed count data.

REMARK.– The same model is obtained by setting $U_i \sim G(\mu_i, \nu)$ and $Z_i|U_i \sim \mathcal{P}(U_i)$. □

REMARK.– To establish a regression model for Z_i, we define $g(\mu_i) = \beta^\top \mathbf{X}_i$. Since $\mu_i > 0$, we typically choose $\ln(\mu_i) = \beta^\top \mathbf{X}_i$ (the log link function). We will return to this point in the next remark below. □

If κ is known, then the negative binomial regression model is a generalized linear model. In R, we can therefore estimate it with the glm function. If κ is unknown, which is usually the case in applied contexts, then we can use the glm.nb function from the MASS package [VEN 02]. This function estimates the parameters β and κ by maximizing the likelihood. By Example 2.5 from section 2.1.2, the likelihood can be written as follows (with the log link function):

$$
L_n(\beta, \kappa) = \prod_{i=1}^{n} \exp\left(Z_i \ln\left(\frac{\kappa e^{\beta^\top \mathbf{X}_i}}{1 + \kappa e^{\beta^\top \mathbf{X}_i}} \right) - \frac{1}{\kappa} \ln(1 + \kappa e^{\beta^\top \mathbf{X}_i}) \right.
$$
$$
\left. + \ln \Gamma\left(Z_i + \frac{1}{\kappa} \right) - \ln\left((Z_i!)\Gamma\left(\frac{1}{\kappa} \right) \right) \right).
$$

We can calculate the likelihood equations by differentiating $\ln L_n(\beta, \kappa)$ with respect to β and κ. For β, we obtain the following equations:

$$
\sum_{i=1}^{n} X_{ij} \left(\frac{Z_i - \mu_i}{1 + \kappa \mu_i} \right) = 0, \quad j = 1, \ldots, p. \tag{3.7}
$$

We note that the parameter κ appears in these equations. The score equation for κ also involves the digamma function (the derivative of $\ln \Gamma(\cdot)$). We will not discuss this score equation any further here, other than mentioning that it involves the parameter β; interested readers can find more information in [HIL 11]. Estimating β and κ therefore alternates between i) estimating β for fixed κ and ii) estimating κ for fixed β. For fixed κ, β is estimated by the usual methods for generalized linear models. Steps i) and ii) are repeated until consecutive approximations of the two parameters converge.

The maximum likelihood estimators of β and κ are consistent and asymptotically Gaussian, which allows us to perform asymptotic inference on β as usual. Readers interested in exploring this further can refer to [CAM 98, HIL 11].

REMARK.– In the negative binomial regression model, we typically use the log link function, which is distinct from the canonical link function in this case. If we use the canonical link function, then the constraint $\mu_i > 0$ would impose that $\beta^\top \mathbf{X}_i < 0$, which restricts the estimates of β. Instead, the log link function is typically preferred, similar to Poisson regression. Equation [2.6] states the score equations of a generalized linear model with an arbitrary link function:

$$\sum_{i=1}^{n} X_{ij} \frac{(Z_i - \mu_i)}{V(\mu_i)} \frac{\partial \mu_i}{\partial \eta_i} = 0, \quad j = 1, \ldots, p.$$

For a negative binomial regression model with the log link function, we have $\partial \mu_i / \partial \eta_i = \mu_i$. Since $V(\mu_i) = \mu_i(1 + \kappa \mu_i)$, we also have:

$$\sum_{i=1}^{n} X_{ij} \frac{(Z_i - \mu_i)}{V(\mu_i)} \frac{\partial \mu_i}{\partial \eta_i} = \sum_{i=1}^{n} X_{ij} \frac{(Z_i - \mu_i)}{\mu_i(1 + \kappa \mu_i)} \mu_i$$

$$= \sum_{i=1}^{n} X_{ij} \left(\frac{Z_i - \mu_i}{1 + \kappa \mu_i} \right).$$

Thus, we recover equation [3.7], as expected.   □

3.3.1. *The NB1 and NB2 variance functions*

The variance in equation [3.6] is a quadratic function in μ_i. Because of this, the negative binomial model described above is sometimes called the "NB2" model [CAM 98, HIL 11]; the "2" refers to the (quadratic) exponent of μ_i in equation [3.6].

Another parameterization of the variance function is also commonly used, obtained by setting $U_i \sim G(\mu_i, \phi\mu_i)$ and $Z_i | U_i \sim \mathcal{P}(U_i)$, with $\phi > 0$. We can find the distribution of Z_i as before by calculating:

$$\mathbb{P}(Z_i = z) = \int_0^\infty e^{-u} \frac{u^z}{z!} \frac{1}{\Gamma(\phi\mu_i)} \phi^{\phi\mu_i} u^{\phi\mu_i - 1} e^{-\phi u} \, du, \quad z = 0, 1, 2, \ldots$$

The details of the calculation are omitted here. The result is a negative binomial distribution with mean:

$$\mathbb{E}(Z_i) = \mu_i$$

and variance:

$$\mathrm{var}(Z_i) = \mu_i \left(1 + \frac{1}{\phi} \right).$$

With this parameterization, the variance is a linear function of μ_i. Accordingly, this model is called the NB1 model [CAM 98, HIL 11]. The regression model is constructed by setting $\mu_i = e^{\beta^\top \mathbf{X}_i}$.

REMARK.– In the NB1 model, the ratio $\mathrm{var}(Z_i)/\mathbb{E}(Z_i)$ is equal to $1 + \frac{1}{\phi}$ for all i. This model therefore describes a form of overdispersion that is constant over all individuals. By contrast, in the NB2 model, the ratio depends on μ_i. □

3.3.2. *Overdispersion tests*

Various overdispersion tests have been proposed in the literature. We will present three of them here. Two are implemented by the `dispersiontest` function from the AER package [KLE 08], and the third can be performed using the `odTest` function from the `pscl` package [JAC 15]. Interested readers can find more information by reading [CAM 98, HIL 11].

We recall that $V(\mu)$ denotes the variance function. For the first two statistics, the overdispersion test is phrased as follows: we test the null hypothesis $H_0 : V(\mu_i) = \mu_i$ against the alternative hypothesis $H_1 : V(\mu_i) = \mu_i + \kappa\mu_i^p$ (with $p = 1$ for the first statistic and $p = 2$ for the second).

If $\kappa = 0$, the data are equidispersed (hypothesis H_0). If $\kappa > 0$, the data are overdispersed. If $\kappa < 0$, they are underdispersed. We can therefore test for overdispersion by testing $H_0 : \kappa = 0$ against $H_1 : \kappa > 0$.

First, consider the alternative hypothesis $\omega_i = V(\mu_i) = \mu_i + \kappa\mu_i$. Under this alternative hypothesis, we have:

$$\frac{\omega_i - \mu_i}{\mu_i} = \kappa.$$

The idea is to fit a Poisson model to the data while estimating μ_i by $\hat{\mu}_i = e^{\hat{\beta}_n^{\top} \mathbf{X}_i}$ and $(\omega_i - \mu_i)/\mu_i$ by:

$$W_i = \frac{(Z_i - \hat{\mu}_i)^2 - Z_i}{\hat{\mu}_i},$$

then estimate the linear model $W_i = \kappa + \epsilon_i$ and finally test whether κ is equal to zero by applying a Wald test (whose statistic asymptotically follows the distribution $\mathcal{N}(0, 1)$ under H_0) [CAM 98].

Under the alternative hypothesis $\omega_i = V(\mu_i) = \mu_i + \kappa\mu_i^2$, we have that:

$$\frac{\omega_i - \mu_i}{\mu_i} = \kappa\mu_i.$$

The idea of this test is similar to the case $p = 1$. Here, we are testing the nullity of κ in the linear model $W_i = \kappa\mu_i + \epsilon_i$ [CAM 98].

The third test is a likelihood-ratio test that views the Poisson model as a special case of the NB2 model when $\kappa = 0$. To test $H_0 : \kappa = 0$, we define the statistic:

$$LRT = 2(\ell_n(\hat{\beta}_n, \hat{\kappa}_n) - \ell_n(\hat{\beta}_n)), \tag{3.8}$$

where $\ell_n(\hat{\beta}_n, \hat{\kappa}_n)$ and $\ell_n(\hat{\beta}_n)$ denote the maximum log-likelihoods of the NB2 and Poisson models, respectively.

Under H_0 (i.e. assuming a Poisson model), the asymptotic distribution of LRT is a mixture $\frac{1}{2}\delta_0 + \frac{1}{2}\chi_1^2$ of the χ^2 distribution with one degree of freedom and the Dirac point mass at zero [CAM 98]. This unusual distribution arises because the parameter κ of the negative binomial model is necessarily strictly positive. To test H_0 to an asymptotic significance level of α, the critical threshold is given by the quantile of order $1 - 2\alpha$ of χ_1^2.

3.4. Application to the NMES1988 data

Let us now return to the NMES1988 data. Figure 3.2 suggests that there is overdispersion in the ofp variable (number of office visits to a physician). The empirical variance/empirical mean ratio of the observations of ofp allows us to roughly quantify this overdispersion:

```
var(ofp)/mean(ofp)
[1] 7.912013
```

The result appears to confirm the presence of overdispersion. A more refined measurement can be performed by estimating:

$$\phi = \frac{\text{var}(Z_i|\mathbf{X}_i)}{\mathbb{E}(Z_i|\mathbf{X}_i)}$$

after fitting the Poisson model in equation [2.17] to the observations. We recall that ϕ can be estimated by:

$$\widehat{\phi} = \frac{1}{n-p} \sum_{i=1}^{n} \frac{(Z_i - \hat{\mu}_i)^2}{\hat{\mu}_i}.$$

The $(Z_i - \hat{\mu}_i)/\sqrt{\hat{\mu}_i}$, $i = 1, \ldots, n$ are known as the Pearson residuals. They can be calculated directly by running the residuals function:

```
fit_pois=glm(ofp~health1+health2+numchron+age+gender+
    fstatus+school+income+med,family=poisson)
p.res=residuals(fit_pois,"pearson")
phi=sum(p.res^2)/df.residual(fit_pois)
phi
[1] 7.006586
```

Although taking into account the explanatory variables success in reducing the overdispersion, there still remains a large and significant amount of overdispersion, as shown by the tests performed in section 3.3.2. The following code implements the Wald test for overdispersion based on the linear variance function $V(\mu_i) = \mu_i + \kappa\mu_i$ (the parameter κ is denoted α in the output of the dispersiontest function):

```
dispersiontest(fit_pois,trafo=1)  # linear parametrization
```

```
               Overdispersion test

data:   fit_pois
z = 11.53, p-value < 2.2e-16
alternative hypothesis: true alpha is greater than 0
sample estimates:
   alpha
5.997146
```

The estimated value of α is approximately 6, so $V(\mu_i) \approx 7\mu_i$, which recovers the value of $\hat{\phi}$ found earlier. The value of the Wald statistic testing $H_0 : \alpha = 0$ against $H_1 : \alpha > 0$ is $z = 11.53$, and its p-value confirms the presence of overdispersion.

The values of $\hat{\alpha}$ and z can be found by running the following code to implement the simple linear regression $W_i = \alpha + \epsilon_i$:

```
mu.est=predict(fit_pois,type="response")

W=((ofp-mu.est)^2-ofp)/mu.est
z.test=lm(W~1)
summary(z.test)
```

This returns the result:

```
Coefficients:
            Estimate  Std. Error  t value  Pr(>|t|)
(Intercept)   5.9971      0.5201    11.53   <2e-16 ***
---
Signif.codes: 0 '***' 0.001 '**' 0.01 '*' 0.05 '.' 0.1 ' ' 1
```

"Intercept" gives us $\hat{\alpha}$, and "t value" gives us z. The test based on the quadratic variance function $V(\mu_i) = \mu_i + \kappa\mu_i^2$ can be performed by running the code:

```
dispersiontest(fit_pois,trafo=2) # quadratic
    parametrization
```

which returns:

```
          Overdispersion test

data:   fit_pois
z = 11.279, p-value < 2.2e-16
alternative hypothesis: true alpha is greater than 0
sample estimates:
      alpha
0.9549329
```

This leads to the same conclusions as before. We note that we can also find the values $\hat{\alpha} = 0.95493$ and $z = 11.28$ by programming the linear model $W_i = \alpha\mu_i + \epsilon_i$ as follows:

```
W=((ofp-mu.est)^2-ofp)/mu.est
z.test=lm(W~0+mu.est)
summary(z.test)
```

This gives:

```
Coefficients:
        Estimate Std. Error t value Pr(>|t|)
mu.est   0.95493    0.08467   11.28   <2e-16 ***
---
Signif. codes: 0 '***' 0.001 '**' 0.01 '*' 0.05 '.' 0.1 '
    ' 1
```

The next step is to fit the quasi-Poisson model to the data:

```
fit_qpois=glm(ofp~health1+health2+numchron+age+gender+
    fstatus+school+income+med,family=quasipoisson)
summary(fit_qpois)
```

The results of fitting are shown below:

```
Coefficients:
             Estimate Std. Error t value Pr(>|t|)
(Intercept)  1.3122787  0.2220627    5.909 3.69e-09 ***
health1      0.2924138  0.0463958    6.303 3.21e-10 ***
health2     -0.3816147  0.0802943   -4.753 2.07e-06 ***
numchron     0.1680809  0.0118317   14.206  < 2e-16 ***
age         -0.0394920  0.0275170   -1.435   0.1513
gender       0.0849809  0.0374750    2.268   0.0234 *
fstatus     -0.0201113  0.0386200   -0.521   0.6026
school       0.0349712  0.0049589    7.052 2.04e-12 ***
income       0.0002906  0.0058890    0.049   0.9606
med          0.1179474  0.0579536    2.035   0.0419 *
---
Signif. codes: 0 '***' 0.001 '**' 0.01 '*' 0.05 '.' 0.1 '
   ' 1

(Dispersion parameter for quasipoisson family taken to be
   7.006754)

    Null deviance: 26943  on 4405  degrees of freedom
Residual deviance: 23933  on 4396  degrees of freedom
AIC: NA

Number of Fisher Scoring iterations: 5
```

The estimated dispersion parameter is 7.006754 (this is the same as the value of $\hat{\phi}$ found above up to rounding errors). As expected, the estimates of the β_j are the same as those obtained with the Poisson model.

However, the "standard errors" are not the same: the standard deviation estimates found by the Poisson model are multiplied by a factor of $\sqrt{7.006754}$.

The following code verifies numerically that $\text{var}(\hat{\beta}_n^Q) = \hat{\phi}\text{var}(\hat{\beta}_n)$:

```
phi=summary(fit_qpois)$dispersion # returns the estimated
    dispersion parameter
cbind(diag(vcov(fit_qpois)),phi*diag(vcov(fit_pois)))
```

Observe that the two columns ($\text{var}(\hat{\beta}_n^Q)$ on the left, $\hat{\phi}\text{var}(\hat{\beta}_n)$ on the right) coincide:

```
                 [,1]            [,2]
(Intercept)  4.931182e-02  4.931182e-02
health1      2.152570e-03  2.152570e-03
health2      6.447170e-03  6.447170e-03
numchron     1.399892e-04  1.399892e-04
age          7.571836e-04  7.571836e-04
gender       1.404373e-03  1.404373e-03
fstatus      1.491501e-03  1.491501e-03
school       2.459099e-05  2.459099e-05
income       3.468033e-05  3.468033e-05
med          3.358625e-03  3.358625e-03
```

As expected, the p-values of the Wald tests are larger in the quasi-Poisson model than in the Poisson model. In particular, the age variable, which was significant in the Poisson model (p-value $= 0.000145$), is no longer significant in the quasi-Poisson model (p-value $= 0.1513$).

Finally, since the quasi-Poisson model is not based on a likelihood, note that the AIC cannot be calculated; this is why the output states "AIC: NA" for "not available."

We can also fit a negative binomial regression model using the glm.nb function from the MASS package [VEN 02] (the differences between models are discussed below). This function has the following syntax (the log link function is selected by default):

```
fit_nb=glm.nb(ofp~health1+health2+numchron+age+gender+
    fstatus+school+income+med)
```

The above line of code returns the output:

```
Coefficients:
              Estimate Std. Error z value Pr(>|z|)
(Intercept)   1.089375   0.206556   5.274 1.33e-07 ***
health1       0.331091   0.049016   6.755 1.43e-11 ***
health2      -0.375657   0.061934  -6.065 1.32e-09 ***
numchron      0.193646   0.012145  15.945  < 2e-16 ***
age          -0.019488   0.025624  -0.761  0.44695
gender        0.091158   0.034557   2.638  0.00834 **
fstatus      -0.024454   0.036076  -0.678  0.49787
school        0.037063   0.004532   8.178 2.90e-16 ***
```

```
income          0.001992    0.005605    0.355  0.72230
med             0.080823    0.057037    1.417  0.15647
---
Signif. codes: 0 '***' 0.001 '**' 0.01 '*' 0.05 '.' 0.1 '
    ' 1

(Dispersion parameter for Negative Binomial(1.153) family
    taken to be 1)

    Null deviance: 5570.6  on 4405  degrees of freedom
Residual deviance: 5041.3  on 4396  degrees of freedom
AIC: 24510

Number of Fisher Scoring iterations: 1


                Theta:  1.1530
            Std. Err.:  0.0316

  2 x log-likelihood:  -24488.1990
```

The line "Theta:1.1530" gives the estimated value of the θ parameter in the expression of the variance $\mathrm{var}(Z_i) = \mu_i + \frac{1}{\theta}\mu_i^2$ used by the NB2 model. Note that we can fix its value (denoted t below) by calling the glm function with the option "family=negative.binomial(t)."

We can test the Poisson model against the NB2 negative binomial model using the likelihood-ratio statistic from Equation [3.8], which is implemented by the odTest function:

```
odTest(fit_nb)
```

This returns the output:

```
Likelihood ratio test of H0: Poisson, as restricted NB
    model:
n.b., the distribution of the test-statistic under H0 is
    non-standard

Critical value of test statistic at the alpha=0.05 level:
    2.7055
Chi-Square Test Statistic=12220.5284 p-value =<2.2e-16
```

As mentioned earlier, the critical threshold of a test with an asymptotic significance level of 0.05 is the quantile of order $1 - 2 \times 0.05 = 0.9$ of the χ_1^2 distribution, which is 2.7055. The result of this test very strongly supports the negative binomial model over the Poisson model.

The test statistic can be reprogrammed as follows:

```
LRT=2*(logLik(fit_nb)-logLik(fit_pois))
LRT
```

This gives:

```
'log Lik.' 12220.53 (df=11)
```

REMARK.– At the end of Chapter 2, we used various functions (lrtest, waldtest, stepAIC, etc.) to construct likelihood-ratio tests, perform automatic selection of variables, and so on in the Poisson model. The same functions can also be used after loading glm.nb.   □

Earlier, we introduced the "sandwich" approach, which allows us to estimate the asymptotic variance of $\hat{\beta}_n^Q$ without making any assumptions about the nature of the ω_i. In R, we can take advantage of an estimator of this type by using the sandwich function from the sandwich package [ZEI 04, ZEI 06].

The following code displays the standard errors calculated by the various methods discussed above (Poisson, quasi-Poisson, negative binomial and sandwich estimators) for each of the β_j of the model in equation [2.17]:

```
nmes.SE=sqrt(cbind(
pois=diag(vcov(fit_pois)),
sand=diag(sandwich(fit_pois)),
qpois=diag(vcov(fit_qpois)),
nbin=diag(vcov(fit_nb))))

round(nmes.SE,4)
```

This gives the table:

	pois	sand	qpois	nbin
(Intercept)	0.0839	0.2188	0.2221	0.2066
health1	0.0175	0.0552	0.0464	0.0490
health2	0.0303	0.0779	0.0803	0.0619
numchron	0.0045	0.0121	0.0118	0.0121
age	0.0104	0.0269	0.0275	0.0256
gender	0.0142	0.0380	0.0375	0.0346
fstatus	0.0146	0.0381	0.0386	0.0361
school	0.0019	0.0054	0.0050	0.0045
income	0.0022	0.0055	0.0059	0.0056
med	0.0219	0.0533	0.0580	0.0570

Here, the standard errors found by the quasi-Poisson model, the negative binomial model and the sandwich approach are relatively close. One advantage of the negative binomial model is that it supports methods of automatic selection of variables, since its fitting is based on a likelihood, unlike the quasi-Poisson and sandwich approaches. This also allows us to predict the response variable of a new individual in terms of its covariables.

In [FRI 16], the authors visualize the mean–variance relation estimated by each of the quasi-Poisson and negative binomial methods graphically to help select the most relevant model.

Their technique is similar to the method used to generate Figure 3.2: i) estimate β in the negative binomial model and then compute $\hat{\mu}_i = e^{\hat{\beta}_n^\top \mathbf{X}_i}$, $i = 1, \ldots, n$; ii) rearrange $\hat{\mu}_1, \ldots, \hat{\mu}_n$ by increasing order and segment the range of values thus obtained into N disjoint intervals (e.g. using the quantiles of $\hat{\mu}_i$); and iii) compute the empirical mean and variance of the response variable (which in our case is ofp) within each interval. This gives N pairs (empirical mean, empirical variance) that can be plotted in the plane and superimposed with the variance functions estimated by each model.

The following code estimates the negative binomial and quasi-Poisson models. Running the command "summary(fit_qpois)$dispersion" returns the value of $\hat{\phi}$.

```
fit_nb=glm.nb(ofp~health1+health2+numchron+age+gender+
    fstatus+school+income+med)

fit_qpois=glm(ofp~health1+health2+numchron+age+gender+
    fstatus+school+income+med,family=quasipoisson)
phi=summary(fit_qpois)$dispersion
```

Next, we construct $N = 100$ pairs (empirical mean, empirical variance) as described above (only the first six are shown).

```
f.nb=fitted(fit_nb,type="response")
intervalle=cut(f.nb,breaks=quantile(f.nb,seq(0,1,by=0.01)
    ))
moy.emp=tapply(ofp,intervalle,mean)
var.emp=tapply(ofp,intervalle,var)
head(cbind(moy.emp,var.emp))
```

```
              moy.emp    var.emp
(1.76,2.52]  1.522727   5.511099
(2.52,2.74]  1.727273   8.482030
(2.74,2.9]   1.886364   8.847252
(2.9,3.05]   3.000000  19.441860
(3.05,3.15]  3.068182   8.716173
(3.15,3.26]  4.500000  98.302326
```

The next step is to plot the set of N points in the plane (Figure 3.4) and superimpose the lines $y = x$, $y = \hat{\phi}x$ and the curve $y = x + \frac{1}{\hat{\theta}}x^2$ representing the variance functions of the Poisson, quasi-Poisson, and NB2 models respectively ($\hat{\theta}$ is returned by the command fit_nb$theta). The mean-variance relation is also estimated by performing a local regression using the lowess function in R.

```
plot(moy.emp,var.emp,xlab="Mean", ylab="Variance", main="
    Mean-variance relation",pch=20)
x = seq(min(moy.emp)-0.5,max(moy.emp)+0.5,0.01)
lines(x,x,col="grey",lwd=2)
lines(x,x*phi,col="red",lwd=2)
lines(x,x+x^2*1/fit_nb$theta,col="blue",lwd=2,lty=2)
lines(lowess(moy.emp,var.emp),col="black",lwd=2,lty=3)
```

```
legend("topleft",lty=c(1,1,2,3),col=c("grey","red","blue"
    ,"black"),lwd=c(2,2,2,2),legend=c("Poisson","quasi-
    Poisson","negative binomial","local regression"),inset
    =0.05)
```

The variance functions of the quasi-Poisson and negative binomial models are close until the mean reaches values of approximately 8. Beyond this point, Figure 3.4 suggests that the quadratic variance function of the negative binomial model gives a better fit.

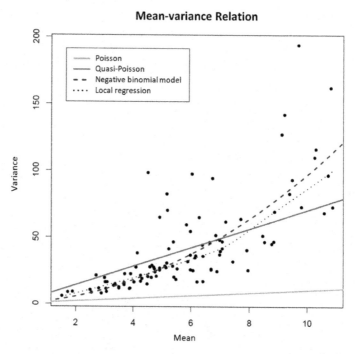

Figure 3.4. *The mean-variance relation estimated by the Poisson, quasi-Poisson, and negative binomial models, as well as by local regression. For a color version of the figure, please see www.iste.co.uk/dupuy/countdata.zip*

4

Count Data and Zero Inflation

This chapter considers one of the causes of overdispersion: zero inflation. This phenomenon, which we will define more precisely later, arises when an "excessive" number of zeros are observed in count data. There are several ways to model this type of data. We will consider a class of models known as "zero-inflated models," which are formulated as mixtures of a Dirac mass and a classical count model (typically, a Poisson model, a generalized Poisson model, a binomial model, etc.).

4.1. Introduction

4.1.1. Zero-inflated models

Consider again the NMES1988 data from the national survey of medical expenditure performed in the USA from 1987 to 1988. The frequency distribution of the ofp variable (representing the number of office visits to a physician; see section 2.6) can be visualized as a bar graph. The following code:

```
visits.fac=factor(ofp,levels=0:max(ofp))
visits.tab=table(visits.fac)
barplot(visits.tab,xlab="Number of office visits to a
    physician",ylab="Frequency",col="lightblue")
```

returns Figure 4.1. In the graph, we can clearly see that the value zero was observed very frequently. This phenomenon is very common in medical and economic studies on healthcare consumption. One interpretation is that there are two different types of zero coexisting in the data. The first type of zero represents individuals who are prepared to visit a physician but never needed to during the period considered by the study. These zeros can be described by a "random regime"; in other words, they can be viewed as the realizations of a random phenomenon that can be modeled by a classical count model with both zero and non-zero values. The second type of zero represents individuals who have systematically decided never to visit a physician. Zeros of the first type are sometimes described as "circumstantial" (see [STA 13]). Zeros of the second type are said to be "structural" [STA 13]; they coexist with the zeros resulting from a classical count model.

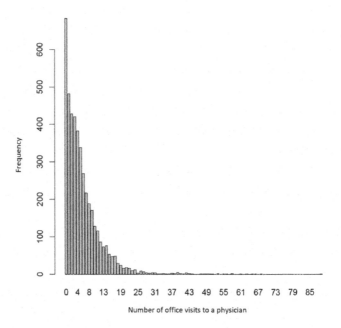

Figure 4.1. *Distribution of the frequency of the number of office visits to a physician (o f p)*

REMARK.– As noted above, the phenomenon of zero inflation is very common in economic studies on healthcare consumption and renunciation. Examples of response variables from these areas that feature zero inflation include: the number of times that an individual visits a physician over a given period of time (for example, see the articles [YEN 01, SAR 06, SAR 09, PIZ 11, STA 13, DIA 7a]); the number of medical prescriptions received by the members of a household over a given period of time (see [STR 99]), the number of times that an individual takes medical leave following a work-related injury (see [CAM 02]).

Zero inflation doesn't only occur in healthcare economics. For example, in car insurance, zero inflation may be observed in the number of at-fault accidents declared by the individuals in an insurance portfolio. An observed zero (no at-fault incidents declared over the course of a year) might fall under either one of the following two cases: i) the insured individual did not experience any incidents; ii) the insured individual was responsible for an incident but chose not to declare it. Individuals can be motivated to avoid declaring an incident by the no-claims system; they may feel that it is preferable to cover the cost of the repairs themselves rather than lose their no-claims bonus. As a result, the number of individuals with no claims over a year is inflated (e.g. relative to a Poisson model) (see [VAS 09, CHA 12]).

Recently, quantitative analyses of international relations and in particular studies of conflict and terrorism have also inspired further research into modeling zero-inflated count data [PIA 11, SAN 14, BAG 15].   □

The term "zero inflation" describes a situation in which the number of zeros observed in a sample of count data is higher than the number predicted by "classical" count models (such as Poisson or binomial models). One of the most common approaches to working with this type of data is to assume that the probability distribution of the count variable (denoted as Z below) is a mixture of a degenerate distribution at zero (i.e. a distribution that takes the value 0 with probability 1) and a count model. To illustrate this idea, we suppose that the count model follows a Poisson distribution $\mathcal{P}(\lambda)$. The distribution of Z can then be written as follows:

$$Z \sim \pi\delta_0 + (1 - \pi)\mathcal{P}(\lambda). \tag{4.1}$$

In the above expression, π is the probability that Z is systematically equal to zero (called the "zero inflation probability" below) and δ_0 denotes the degenerate distribution at zero. Equation [4.1] can alternatively be interpreted as follows:

$$Z \sim \begin{cases} 0 & \text{with probability } \pi \\ \mathcal{P}(\lambda) & \text{with probability } 1 - \pi \end{cases} \tag{4.2}$$

The event $\{Z = 0\}$ can therefore arise from two different situations, one for each of the types of zero identified above. In the first situation, which occurs with probability π, the event $\{Z = 0\}$ is guaranteed. In the second situation, which occurs with probability $1 - \pi$, the zero is observed as the realization of a random experiment, which we have chosen to model by a Poisson distribution here. We write S for a variable that takes the value 1 when the observed zero is structural (first situation) and the value 0 when the observed zero is circumstantial, or "random" (second situation). This variable, which contains information about the type of the observed zero, is not itself observable. It is simply a theoretical formalism that allows us to compute the probability distribution of Z. The distribution of S satisfies $\mathbb{P}(S = 1) = \pi$ and $\mathbb{P}(S = 0) = 1 - \pi$. We can rewrite equation [4.2] by stating that:

– conditional on the event $\{S = 1\}$, Z takes the value 0 with probability 1,

– conditional on the event $\{S = 0\}$, Z takes the value z (for $z = 0, 1, \ldots$) with probability $e^{-\lambda}\frac{\lambda^z}{z!}$. In particular, if S is 0, then Z takes the value 0 with probability $e^{-\lambda}$.

Hence, by the law of total probability, we have that:

$$\mathbb{P}(Z = 0) = \mathbb{P}(Z = 0|S = 1)\mathbb{P}(S = 1) + \mathbb{P}(Z = 0|S = 0)\mathbb{P}(S = 0)$$

$$= 1 \cdot \pi + e^{-\lambda} \cdot (1 - \pi)$$

$$= \pi + (1 - \pi)e^{-\lambda}.$$

Similarly, if $z = 1, 2, \ldots$, we can show that:

$$\mathbb{P}(Z = z) = \mathbb{P}(Z = z|S = 1)\mathbb{P}(S = 1) + \mathbb{P}(Z = z|S = 0)\mathbb{P}(S = 0)$$

$$= 0 \cdot \pi + \frac{e^{-\lambda}\lambda^z}{z!} \cdot (1 - \pi)$$

$$= (1 - \pi)\frac{e^{-\lambda}\lambda^z}{z!}.$$

We can therefore summarize the probability distribution of Z as follows:

$$\mathbb{P}(Z = z) = \begin{cases} \pi + (1 - \pi)e^{-\lambda} & z = 0 \\ (1 - \pi)\frac{e^{-\lambda}\lambda^z}{z!} & z = 1, 2, \ldots \end{cases} \quad [4.3]$$

The model in equation [4.1] is called a zero-inflated Poisson model or ZIP model (denoted as $\text{ZIP}(\lambda, \pi)$ below). When π is equal to zero, the ZIP model reduces to the Poisson distribution with parameter $\lambda > 0$. It is easy to see that $\mathbb{P}(Z = 0) = e^{-\lambda} + \pi(1 - e^{-\lambda})$ is greater than or equal to the probability $e^{-\lambda}$ that a Poisson distribution with parameter λ yields the value zero. In the model from equation [4.1], the latter probability is increased by the extra term $\pi(1 - e^{-\lambda})$.

In R, several packages include functions dedicated to zero-inflated models. The dzipois (VGAM package, see [YEE 16]), dZIP (gamlss package, see [STA 07]) and dzip (extraDistr package, see [WOL 17]) functions each return the probability density function of a ZIP distribution. The syntax of these functions is as follows:

```
dzipois(x,lambda,piz)
dZIP(x,lambda,piz)
dzip(x,lambda,piz)
```

where piz is the zero-inflation probability π. The following code plots the probability density functions of a Poisson distribution $\mathcal{P}(\lambda)$ and a ZIP model $\text{ZIP}(\lambda, \pi)$ as bar graphs (see Figure 4.2):

```
par(mfrow=c(1,2))

x=0:10; lambda=3

piz=0.2 # zero inflation probability
barplot(rbind(dzipois(x,lambda,piz), dpois(x,lambda)),
    beside=TRUE,col=c("black","lightgrey"),names.arg=as.
    character(x))

piz=0.7 # zero inflation probability
barplot(rbind(dzipois(x,lambda,piz), dpois(x,lambda)),
    beside=TRUE,col=c("black","lightgrey"),names.arg=as.
    character(x))
```

The probabilities $\mathbb{P}(\mathcal{P}(3) = x)$ and $\mathbb{P}(\text{ZIP}(3, 0.2) = x)$ (for $x = 0, \ldots, 10$) shown in Figure 4.2 can be calculated as follows:

```
cbind("Poisson"=dpois(x,lambda),"ZIP"=dzipois(x,lambda,
    piz))
```

which returns the table:

```
              Poisson              ZIP
 [1,] 0.0497870684 0.2398296547
 [2,] 0.1493612051 0.1194889641
 [3,] 0.2240418077 0.1792334461
 [4,] 0.2240418077 0.1792334461
 [5,] 0.1680313557 0.1344250846
 [6,] 0.1008188134 0.0806550508
 [7,] 0.0504094067 0.0403275254
 [8,] 0.0216040315 0.0172832252
 [9,] 0.0081015118 0.0064812094
[10,] 0.0027005039 0.0021604031
[11,] 0.0008101512 0.0006481209
```

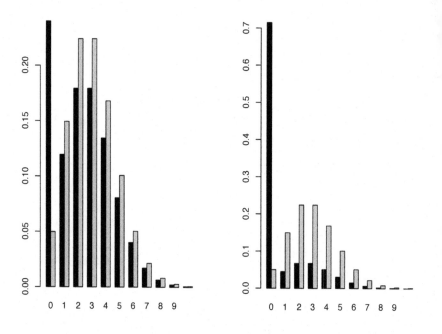

Figure 4.2. *Frequency distributions of two ZIP models (left: ZIP$(3, 0.2)$, right: ZIP$(3, 0.7)$) (black) and a Poisson model ($\lambda = 3$) (gray)*

We may be wondering whether there exists some value of $\mu > 0$ for which the Poisson distribution $\mathcal{P}(\mu)$ has a probability of 0 equal to that of the model ZIP(λ, π). The answer is yes; simply define $\mu = -\ln\left(e^{-\lambda} + \pi(1 - e^{-\lambda})\right)$. To illustrate, Figure 4.3 shows the frequency distributions of ZIP(λ, π), $\mathcal{P}(\lambda)$ and

$\mathcal{P}(\mu)$, for $\lambda = 3$, $\pi = 0.5$ and μ as defined above. This figure was generated using the R code listed below:

```
x=0:10; lambda=3; piz=.5
mu=-log(exp(-lambda)+piz*(1-exp(-lambda)))
barplot(rbind(dzipois(x,lambda,pstr0=piz),dpois(x,mu),
    dpois(x,lambda)),beside=TRUE,col=c("black","lightgrey"
    ,"white"),names.arg=as.character(x))
```

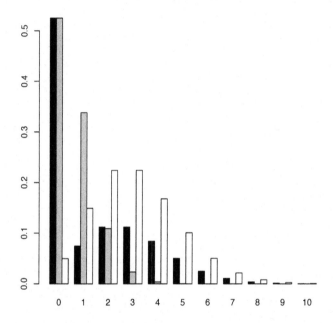

Figure 4.3. *Frequency distributions of the models ZIP(3, 0.5) (black),* $\mathcal{P}(\mu)$ *for* $\mu = -\ln\left(e^{-3} + 0.5\left(1 - e^{-3}\right)\right)$ *(gray) and* $\mathcal{P}(3)$ *(white)*

Consider the Poisson distribution with parameter μ. The probability $e^{-\mu}$ that this distribution takes the value 0 decreases as its mean μ increases. Therefore, although Poisson distributions are not directly incompatible with high probabilities of observing zero, any Poisson distribution with a high probability of 0 necessarily has a relatively small mean. Figure 4.3 illustrates this observation, showing that the distribution $\mathcal{P}(\mu)$ only takes values greater than or equal to 3 with very low probability. The effective support of the distribution $\mathcal{P}(3)$, on the contrary, ranges over a wider set of values, but cannot correctly describe the zero inflation. The model $\mathrm{ZIP}(3, 0.5)$ can be viewed as a compromise that satisfies two requirements that are contradictory for a Poisson distribution: a high probability of observing the value 0 and an expected value that is not "too small".

REMARK.– From equation [4.3], we can easily compute the mean and variance of the random variable $Z \sim \pi\delta_0 + (1 - \pi)\mathcal{P}(\lambda)$. We have:

$$\mathbb{E}(Z) = \sum_{z=0}^{+\infty} z\mathbb{P}(Z = z)$$

$$= (1 - \pi)\sum_{z=0}^{+\infty} z\frac{e^{-\lambda}\lambda^z}{z!}$$

$$= (1 - \pi)\lambda,$$

since $\mathbb{E}(\mathcal{P}(\lambda)) = \sum_{z=0}^{+\infty} z\frac{e^{-\lambda}\lambda^z}{z!} = \lambda$, and:

$$\text{var}(Z) = \sum_{z=0}^{+\infty}(1 - \pi)z^2\frac{e^{-\lambda}\lambda^z}{z!} - [(1 - \pi)\lambda]^2$$

$$= (1 - \pi)\left(\lambda + \lambda^2\right) - [(1 - \pi)\lambda]^2$$

$$= (1 + \pi\lambda)(1 - \pi)\lambda$$

$$= (1 + \pi\lambda)\mathbb{E}(Z).$$

Whenever the zero inflation probability π is strictly positive, it can be easily seen that $\text{var}(Z) > \mathbb{E}(Z)$. Hence, zero inflation necessarily leads to overdispersion in the distribution of Z (we recall that the Poisson distribution is equidispersed, i.e. $\text{var}(Z) = \mathbb{E}(Z)$).   □

The expression in equation [4.1] defines a zero-inflated Poisson model. Other zero-inflated models can be defined by replacing this Poisson distribution by other count models (e.g. a binomial distribution or a negative binomial distribution). We write $\mathcal{B}(m, p)$ for the binomial distribution with parameters (m, p), where $m \in \{1, 2, \ldots\}$ and $p \in (0, 1)$. The zero-inflated binomial (ZIB) model is defined as follows:

$$Z \sim \pi\delta_0 + (1 - \pi)\mathcal{B}(m, p),$$

or, alternatively as:

$$Z \sim \begin{cases} 0 & \text{with probability } \pi \\ \mathcal{B}(m,p) & \text{with probability } 1 - \pi \end{cases}$$

We write $\text{ZIB}(m, p, \pi)$ for this model. After performing a few simple calculations, the probability distribution of Z is given by:

$$\mathbb{P}(Z = z) = \begin{cases} \pi + (1 - \pi)(1 - p)^m & z = 0 \\ (1 - \pi)C_m^z p^z (1 - p)^{m-z} & z = 1, 2, \ldots, m \end{cases}$$

REMARK.– From these expressions, we can easily show that $\mathbb{E}(Z) = (1 - \pi)mp$ and $\text{var}(Z) = (1 - \pi)mp[1 - p(1 - m\pi)]$. $\square$

The dzibinom (VGAM package, see [YEE 16]), dZIBI (gamlss package, see [STA 07]) and dzib (package extraDistr, see [WOL 17]) functions return the probability density function of a ZIB distribution. The syntax of these functions is as follows:

```
dzibinom(x,m,p,piz)
dZIBI(x,m,p,piz)
dzib(x,m,p,piz)
```

The following code implements the probability density functions of the distributions $\text{ZIB}(10, 0.4, 0.5)$ and $\mathcal{B}(10, 0.4)$ (see Figure 4.4):

```
p=0.4; m=10; x=0:m
piz=0.5  # zero inflation probability
barplot(rbind(dzibinom(x,m,p,piz),dbinom(x,m,p)),beside=
    TRUE,col=c("black","lightgrey"),names.arg=as.character
    (x))
```

The probabilities associated with them can be accessed with the command:

```
cbind("binomial"=dbinom(x,m,p),"ZIB"=dzibinom(x,m,p,piz))
```

which returns the following table:

```
               binomial              ZIB
 [1,]  0.0060466176  0.5030233088
 [2,]  0.0403107840  0.0201553920
 [3,]  0.1209323520  0.0604661760
 [4,]  0.2149908480  0.1074954240
 [5,]  0.2508226560  0.1254113280
 [6,]  0.2006581248  0.1003290624
 [7,]  0.1114767360  0.0557383680
 [8,]  0.0424673280  0.0212336640
 [9,]  0.0106168320  0.0053084160
[10,]  0.0015728640  0.0007864320
[11,]  0.0001048576  0.0000524288
```

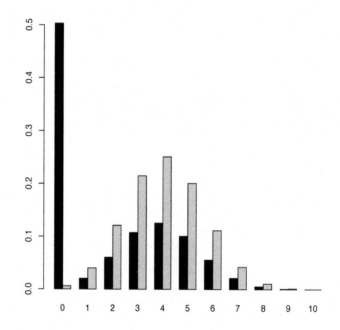

Figure 4.4. *Frequency distributions of the ZIB model ZIB*$(10, 0.4, 0.5)$
(black) and the binomial model $\mathcal{B}(10, 0.4)$ *(gray)*

REMARK.– As before, we can determine a value of q for the distribution $\mathcal{B}(m, q)$ such that the probability of observing zero is equal for both $\mathcal{B}(m, q)$ and ZIB(m, p, π). If m, p and π are fixed, then we can simply take q such that $\pi + (1 - \pi)(1 - p)^m = (1 - q)^m$, which gives

$q = 1 - (\pi + (1 - \pi)(1 - p)^m)^{1/m}$. Figure 4.5 shows the frequency distributions of ZIB$(10, 0.4, 0.5)$ and $\mathcal{B}(10, q)$.

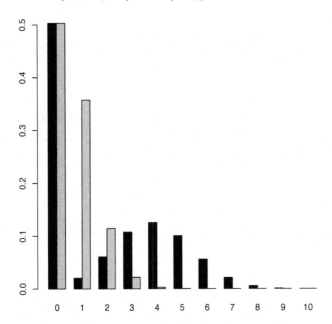

Figure 4.5. *Frequency distributions of the ZIB model ZIB$(10, 0.4, 0.5)$ (black) and the binomial model $\mathcal{B}(10, q)$ for*
$$q = 1 - (0.5 + (1 - 0.5)(1 - 0.4)^{10})^{1/10} \text{ (gray)}$$

We note that the probability of observing values greater than or equal to 4 is low for the $\mathcal{B}(10, q)$ distribution. On the contrary, the $\mathcal{B}(10, 0.4)$ distribution is not capable of describing the zero inflation. Again, the zero-inflated model (here the model ZIB$(10, 0.4, 0.5)$) appears to be more suitable for describing a high probability of observing zero without reducing the effective support of the distribution.   □

As stated in section 2.1, the negative binomial distribution is defined as the probability distribution of the random variable Z that counts the number of failures required before obtaining k successes (for $k \in \{1, 2, \ldots\}$) in a sequence of independent trials with constant probability of success p. Several parameterizations of this distribution are available, for example, using the dnbinom function from the stats package in R. One parameterization expresses the probability density as a function of k (called the "size" in the dnbinom function) and a parameter $\mu > 0$ (this distribution is denoted as $\mathcal{NB}(\mu, k)$ below):

$$\mathbb{P}(Z = z) = C^z_{z+k-1} \left(\frac{\mu}{\mu + k} \right)^z \left(\frac{k}{\mu + k} \right)^k, \quad z = 0, 1, 2, \dots$$

In this case, the probability of success is $p = k/(\mu + k)$. Using $\mathcal{NB}(\mu, k)$, we can define a zero-inflated negative binomial (ZINB) model as follows:

$$Z \sim \pi \delta_0 + (1 - \pi)\mathcal{NB}(\mu, k),$$

or, alternatively:

$$Z \sim \begin{cases} 0 & \text{with probability } \pi \\ \mathcal{NB}(\mu, k) & \text{with probability } 1 - \pi \end{cases}$$

We shall write $\text{ZINB}(\mu, k, \pi)$ for this model. We can find the probability distribution of Z by performing a simple calculation:

$$\mathbb{P}(Z = z) = \begin{cases} \pi + (1 - \pi) \left(\frac{k}{\mu+k} \right)^k & z = 0 \\ (1 - \pi)C^z_{z+k-1} \left(\frac{\mu}{\mu+k} \right)^z \left(\frac{k}{\mu+k} \right)^k & z = 1, 2, \dots \end{cases}$$

The `dzinegbin` function from the `VGAM` package implements the probability density of the distribution $\text{ZINB}(\mu, k, \pi)$. The R code:

```
x=0:13
barplot(rbind(dzinegbin(x,pstr0=0.2,mu=3,size=10),dnbinom
    (x,mu=3,size=10)),beside=TRUE,col=c("black","lightgrey
    "),names.arg=as.character(x))
cbind("neg.binomial"=dnbinom(x,mu=3,size=10),"ZINB"=
    dzinegbin(x,pstr0=0.2,mu=3,size=10))
```

plots the probability densities of $\text{ZINB}(3, 10, 0.2)$ and $\mathcal{NB}(3, 10)$, for $z = 0, 1, \dots, 13$ (see Figure 4.6) and displays the corresponding probability values:

```
        neg.binomial            ZINB
 [1,]   0.0725381503  0.2580305202
 [2,]   0.1673957314  0.1339165851
 [3,]   0.2124638130  0.1699710504
 [4,]   0.1961204427  0.1568963542
 [5,]   0.1470903321  0.1176722656
 [6,]   0.0950429838  0.0760343870
 [7,]   0.0548324906  0.0438659925
 [8,]   0.0289226324  0.0231381059
 [9,]   0.0141832140  0.0113465712
[10,]   0.0065460988  0.0052368790
[11,]   0.0028702125  0.0022961700
[12,]   0.0012042850  0.0009634280
[13,]   0.0004863459  0.0003890767
[14,]   0.0001899339  0.0001519471
```

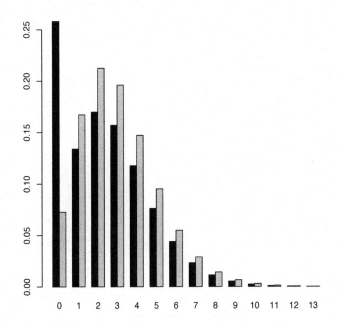

Figure 4.6. *Frequency distributions of the ZINB model ZINB*$(3, 10, 0.2)$
and the negative binomial model $\mathcal{NB}(3, 10)$ *(gray)*

The `dzinb` function from the `extraDistr` package also gives the probability density of a ZINB distribution, this time with a slightly different parameterization:

$$\mathbb{P}(Z = z) = \begin{cases} \pi + (1 - \pi)p^k & z = 0 \\ (1 - \pi)C_{z+k-1}^z (1 - p)^z \, p^k & z = 1, 2, \ldots, \end{cases}$$

where $p = k/(\mu + k)$. The probability distribution of $\text{ZINB}(3, 10, 0.2)$ can therefore also be obtained as follows using `dzinb`:

```
mu=3; size=10; p=size/(mu+size)
dzinb(x,size,p,pi=0.2)
```

Let us return to the parameterization of the `dzinegbin` function. Again, we can find a value of λ for $\mathcal{NB}(\lambda, k)$ such that both the models $\mathcal{NB}(\lambda, k)$ and $\text{ZINB}(\mu, k, \pi)$ have the same probability of observing zero. For fixed μ, k and π, we can simply choose λ such that:

$$\pi + (1 - \pi)\left(\frac{k}{\mu + k}\right)^k = \left(\frac{k}{\lambda + k}\right)^k,$$

which gives:

$$\lambda = k \left(\pi + (1 - \pi)\left(\frac{k}{\mu + k}\right)^k\right)^{-\frac{1}{k}} - k.$$

Figure 4.7 shows the frequency distributions of $\text{ZINB}(3, 10, 0.2)$ and $\mathcal{NB}(\lambda, 10)$, with λ as above.

We note that the probability of observing values greater than or equal to 4 is very small for $\mathcal{NB}(\lambda, 10)$. On the contrary, the model $\mathcal{NB}(3, 10)$ does not properly describe the zero inflation. The zero-inflated model (which here is the model $\text{ZINB}(3, 10, 0.2)$) once again provides a more suitable way of representing the high probability of observing zero without reducing the effective support of the distribution.

REMARK.– An alternative to zero-inflated models is given by the so-called "hurdle" models proposed by [MUL 86]. In a zero-inflated model, each zero is generated by one of the following two mechanisms: i) the mechanism underlying the class of "structural zeros" and ii) the probability distribution of the relevant count model. In a hurdle model, the zeros are generated by a single process and all non-zero observations are managed by a separate process. For instance, the first process can be modeled by a Bernoulli distribution, together with a count model truncated at zero for the second process. These models are not discussed in any further depth in this book. Interested readers can find more information in [CAM 98, WIN 13].   □

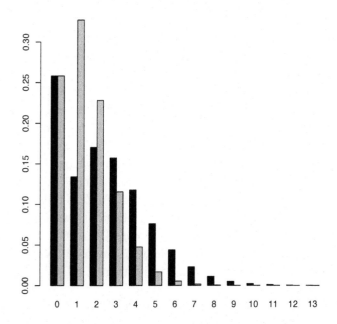

Figure 4.7. *Frequency distributions of the ZINB model ZINB*$(3, 10, 0.2)$ *(black) and the negative binomial model* $\mathcal{NB}(\lambda, 10)$ *(gray)*

So far, we have introduced the concept of zero inflation and explained why classical count models (such as Poisson models, binomial models, or negative binomial models) are unsuitable for representing zero-inflated data. Zero-inflated regression models (and in particular, zero-inflated Poisson (ZIP) regression models and zero-inflated binomial (ZIB) regression models) offer better solutions to the problems associated with zero inflation. These models are described in the next section.

4.1.2. *Zero-inflated regression models*

Zero-inflated models first appeared in the statistical literature in the 1960s (interested readers can find references in [JOH 05]). The model $ZIP(\lambda, \pi)$, with a parameter λ that depends on the explanatory variables (regressors, covariables), was proposed by [MUL 86]. In [LAM 92], the explanatory variables also influence the zero inflation probability π. The models presented by [MUL 86, LAM 92] are therefore zero-inflated Poisson *regression* models. A zero-inflated binomial regression model was later described by [HAL 00].

Since then, various other zero-inflated regression models have been developed, designed for increasingly complex situations (multivariate responses, repeated data, missing or censored data, etc.). A non-exhaustive list of examples might include the zero-inflated generalized Poisson model [FAM 03, GUP 04, FAM 06, CZA 05, CZA 07], zero-inflated regression models with random effects [HAL 00, HAL 04, XIA 07, XIE 09, ZHU 17], the zero-inflated semi-parametric Poisson model [LAM 06, HE 10, FEN 11] and the endpoint-inflated binomial (EIB) model introduced by [DEN 15] to model inflation at both zero and the value m in a sample from the binomial distribution $\mathcal{B}(m, p)$ (see also [TIA 15, DUP 17]). Zero-inflated regression models have also been developed for situations with missing data [CHE 11, LUK 16, DIA 17b] or censored data [PRA 09]. A zero-inflated model for a bivariate response variable was proposed by [WAN 03]. A zero-inflated multinomial regression model is outlined in [DIA 18].

There are several very comprehensive publications that discuss ZIP and ZINB regression models in great detail (see, for example, [CAM 98, WIN 13]; the thesis [ERH 06], written in German, should also be mentioned). The next few sections give a brief description of the ZIP model before focusing on zero-inflated binomial and multinomial regression models.

4.2. ZIP regression model

4.2.1. *Definition*

Suppose that we are observing a count variable Z on a sample of n individuals. Let us write Z_i for the observed value of Z at the i-th individual, $i = 1, \ldots, n$. We can construct a zero-inflated Poisson regression model for Z_i by allowing the probability π and the intensity λ in equation [4.1] to depend on the individual i via the explanatory variables (or *covariables*). This model can be stated as:

$$\mathbb{P}(Z_i = z) = \begin{cases} \pi_i + (1 - \pi_i)e^{-\lambda_i} & z = 0 \\ (1 - \pi_i)\frac{e^{-\lambda_i}\lambda_i^z}{z!} & z = 1, 2, \ldots \end{cases}$$

where π_i and λ_i are, respectively, functions of the vectors of covariables $\mathbf{W}_i = (W_{i1}, \ldots, W_{iq})^\top$ and $\mathbf{X}_i = (X_{i1}, \ldots, X_{ip})^\top$ (setting $X_{i1} = W_{i1} = 1$). The components of these vectors can be either qualitative or quantitative. The probability π_i is usually described by a logistic regression:

$$\text{logit}(\pi_i) = \gamma^\top \mathbf{W}_i = \gamma_1 + \gamma_2 W_{i2} + \ldots + \gamma_q W_{iq}$$

$$\Longleftrightarrow \pi_i = \frac{\exp\left(\gamma^\top \mathbf{W}_i\right)}{1 + \exp\left(\gamma^\top \mathbf{W}_i\right)} \in (0, 1),$$

and the intensity λ_i is usually modeled by:

$$\ln(\lambda_i) = \beta^\top \mathbf{X}_i = \beta_1 + \beta_2 X_{i2} + \ldots + \beta_p X_{ip}$$

$$\Longleftrightarrow \lambda_i = \exp\left(\beta^\top \mathbf{X}_i\right), \tag{4.4}$$

where $\beta = (\beta_1, \ldots, \beta_p)^\top$ and $\gamma = (\gamma_1, \ldots, \gamma_q)^\top$ are vectors of unknown parameters. We can summarize this model in the form:

$$\forall i = 1, \ldots, n, \quad \begin{cases} Z_i \sim \pi_i \delta_0 + (1 - \pi_i)\mathcal{P}(\lambda_i) \\ \text{logit}(\pi_i) = \gamma^\top \mathbf{W}_i \\ \ln(\lambda_i) = \beta^\top \mathbf{X}_i \end{cases} \tag{4.5}$$

Notationally, we write that $Z_i \sim \text{ZIP}(\lambda_i, \pi_i)$. Conditional on $\mathbf{X}_i$ and $\mathbf{W}_i$, the mean and variance of Z_i are, respectively, given by:

$$\mathbb{E}(Z_i | \mathbf{X}_i, \mathbf{W}_i) = (1 - \pi_i)\lambda_i = \frac{\exp\left(\beta^\top \mathbf{X}_i\right)}{1 + \exp\left(\gamma^\top \mathbf{W}_i\right)}$$

and

$$\text{var}(Z_i | \mathbf{X}_i, \mathbf{W}_i) = (1 + \pi_i \lambda_i)(1 - \pi_i)\lambda_i = (1 + \pi_i \lambda_i)\mathbb{E}(Z_i | \mathbf{X}_i, \mathbf{W}_i).$$

The conditional distribution of Z_i is overdispersed, since $(1 + \pi_i \lambda_i) > 1$, and hence $\text{var}(Z_i | \mathbf{X}_i, \mathbf{W}_i) > \mathbb{E}(Z_i | \mathbf{X}_i, \mathbf{W}_i)$.

REMARK.– Similar to classical Poisson regression, we can introduce an exposure term into the model in equation [4.5] if the observation period is not constant for every individual. Let E_i be the observation period of the i-th individual. We arrive at the following model: $Z_i \sim \pi_i \delta_0 + (1 - \pi_i)\mathcal{P}(E_i \cdot \lambda_i)$, i.e. $Z_i \sim \pi_i \delta_0 + (1 - \pi_i)\mathcal{P}(\exp(\ln(E_i) + \beta^\top \mathbf{X}_i))$. The term $\ln(E_i)$ appears as an additional covariable with a known coefficient, equal to 1. □

4.2.2. Estimation in the ZIP model

Suppose that we have a sample $(Z_1, \mathbf{X}_1, \mathbf{W}_1)$, ..., $(Z_n, \mathbf{X}_n, \mathbf{W}_n)$ of independent observations of the model in equation [4.5] (to simplify the notation, we shall omit the exposure term). The parameter $\psi = (\beta^\top, \gamma^\top)^\top$ of the model can be estimated by the maximum likelihood method. The likelihood can be computed as follows:

$$L_n(\psi) = \prod_{i=1}^{n} \left(\pi_i + (1 - \pi_i)e^{-\lambda_i} \right)^{1_{\{Z_i=0\}}} \cdot \left((1 - \pi_i)e^{-\lambda_i}\frac{\lambda_i^{Z_i}}{Z_i!} \right)^{1_{\{Z_i>0\}}}.$$

From this, we can deduce the log-likelihood $\ell_n(\psi) = \ln L_n(\psi)$:

$$\ell_n(\psi) = \sum_{i=1}^{n} 1_{\{Z_i=0\}} \ln \left(\pi_i + (1 - \pi_i)e^{-\lambda_i} \right)$$

$$+ \sum_{i=1}^{n} 1_{\{Z_i>0\}} \left(\ln(1 - \pi_i) - \lambda_i + Z_i \ln \lambda_i - \ln(Z_i!) \right).$$

From equation [4.5], we find:

$$\pi_i + (1 - \pi_i)e^{-\lambda_i} = \frac{\exp\left(\gamma^\top \mathbf{W}_i\right) + \exp\left(-\exp(\beta^\top \mathbf{X}_i)\right)}{1 + \exp\left(\gamma^\top \mathbf{W}_i\right)},$$

which then gives us:

$$\ell_n(\psi) = \sum_{i=1}^{n} 1_{\{Z_i=0\}} \ln \left(\exp\left(\gamma^\top \mathbf{W}_i\right) + \exp\left(-\exp(\beta^\top \mathbf{X}_i)\right) \right)$$

$$+ \sum_{i=1}^{n} 1_{\{Z_i > 0\}} \left(Z_i \beta^\top \mathbf{X}_i - \exp(\beta^\top \mathbf{X}_i) - \ln(Z_i!) \right) \qquad [4.6]$$

$$- \sum_{i=1}^{n} \ln \left(1 + \exp \left(\gamma^\top \mathbf{W}_i \right) \right).$$

The maximum likelihood estimator $\hat{\psi}_n$ of ψ is obtained by solving the following estimation equation (known as the score equation):

$$\frac{\partial}{\partial \psi} \ell_n(\psi) \bigg|_{\psi = \hat{\psi}_n} = 0.$$

This is, in fact, a system of $p + q$ equations obtained by differentiating $\ell_n(\psi)$ with respect to each of the γ_j and the β_j. This estimator does not have an explicit expression. We can approximate it using nonlinear optimization algorithms (such as the Newton–Raphson algorithm). In [LAM 92, HAL 00], the authors apply the expectation–maximization (EM) algorithm to maximize the log-likelihood in equation [4.6]. The following section restates this algorithm for completeness. Readers can safely skip this section without detracting from the rest of the presentation, if they wish.

4.2.2.1. *The EM algorithm*

The EM algorithm, introduced by [DEM 77], is an iterative algorithm that can be used to maximize a likelihood in the presence of missing data. Let S_i be the indicator variable that takes the value 1 if Z_i is equal to 0 with probability 1 and takes the value 0 if Z_i follows the Poisson distribution $\mathcal{P}(\lambda_i)$. In the context of zero inflation, the indicator variables $S_1, \ldots, S_n$ are the missing data. If these variables were observed, the log-likelihood (said to be complete) of the parameter ψ based on the independent sample $(Z_1, S_1, \mathbf{X}_1, \mathbf{W}_1)$, $\ldots$, $(Z_n, S_n, \mathbf{X}_n, \mathbf{W}_n)$ would have the following expression (for detailed calculations, see section 4.2.2.3):

$$\ell_n^c(\psi) = \sum_{i=1}^{n} \left[S_i \gamma^\top \mathbf{W}_i - \ln \left(1 + \exp \left(\gamma^\top \mathbf{W}_i \right) \right) \right]$$

$$+ \sum_{i=1}^{n} (1 - S_i) \left[Z_i \beta^\top \mathbf{X}_i - \exp(\beta^\top \mathbf{X}_i) - \ln(Z_i!) \right]. \qquad [4.7]$$

Of course, we cannot compute this log-likelihood, since the S_i, $i = 1, \ldots, n$, are unobserved. The idea of the EM algorithm is to iterate two steps, the E-step (for expectation) and the M-step (for maximization), until a stopping criterion is satisfied (readers interested in the mathematical basis of this algorithm can find more information from the extremely comprehensive discussion by [MCL 08]). At the $(k + 1)$-th iteration of the algorithm, these steps can be stated as follows:

E-step: Compute the expectation of the complete log-likelihood conditional on the observations $\mathcal{O}_n := \{(Z_1, \mathbf{X}_1, \mathbf{W}_1), \ldots, (Z_n, \mathbf{X}_n, \mathbf{W}_n)\}$ under the distribution with parameter $\psi^{(k)}$ (where $\psi^{(k)}$ denotes the estimate of ψ established by the k-th iteration of the algorithm). Let this expectation be denoted by $\mathbb{E}\left(\ell_n^c(\psi)|\mathcal{O}_n; \psi^{(k)}\right)$.

This step simply requires us to compute the conditional expectation of S_i given the observations under the distribution with parameter $\psi^{(k)}$ (the details of the calculation can be found in section 4.2.2.3). The value of this conditional expectation is as follows:

$$\mathbb{E}(S_i|\mathcal{O}_n; \psi^{(k)}) = \begin{cases} 0 & \text{if } Z_i > 0 \\ \left[1 + \exp\left(-\gamma^{(k)\top}\mathbf{W}_i - \exp\left(\beta^{(k)\top}\mathbf{X}_i\right)\right)\right]^{-1} & \text{if } Z_i = 0 \end{cases}$$

Intuitively, we can view this value as an estimate of the "missing" datapoint S_i. We then substitute this datapoint into equation [4.7] to obtain:

$$\mathbb{E}\left(\ell_n^c(\psi)|\mathcal{O}_n; \psi^{(k)}\right)$$

$$= \sum_{i=1}^n \left[\mathbb{E}(S_i|\mathcal{O}_n; \psi^{(k)})\gamma^\top\mathbf{W}_i - \ln\left(1 + \exp\left(\gamma^\top\mathbf{W}_i\right)\right)\right]$$

$$+ \sum_{i=1}^n (1 - \mathbb{E}(S_i|\mathcal{O}_n; \psi^{(k)}))\left[Z_i\beta^\top\mathbf{X}_i - \exp(\beta^\top\mathbf{X}_i) - \ln(Z_i!)\right]$$

$$:= \tilde{\ell}_{n,1}(\gamma) + \tilde{\ell}_{n,2}(\beta).$$

M-step: Find the value $\psi^{(k+1)}$ that maximizes the function $\psi \mapsto \mathbb{E}(\ell_n^c(\psi)|\mathcal{O}_n; \psi^{(k)})$.

The expression of this function is very convenient for finding $\psi^{(k+1)}$. Indeed, $\mathbb{E}(\ell_n^c(\psi)|\mathcal{O}_n; \psi^{(k)})$ splits into the sum of two terms, one depending on γ, and the other depending on β. Each of the terms $\tilde{\ell}_{n,1}(\gamma)$ and $\tilde{\ell}_{n,2}(\beta)$ can therefore be maximized separately. Furthermore, $\tilde{\ell}_{n,1}(\gamma)$ coincides with the log-likelihood of a logistic regression model (where $\mathbb{E}(S_i|\mathcal{O}_n; \psi^{(k)})$ plays the role of a response variable) with linear predictor $\gamma^\top W_i$. Similarly, $\tilde{\ell}_{n,2}(\beta)$ coincides with the log-likelihood of a Poisson regression model for the Z_i with linear predictor $\beta^\top X_i$. Here, the terms of the log-likelihood are weighted by $(1 - \mathbb{E}(S_i|\mathcal{O}_n; \psi^{(k)}))$, $i = 1, \ldots, n$, which only depend on the value $\psi^{(k)}$. Thus, the M-step essentially reduces to the estimation of two generalized linear models.

The E- and M-steps of the algorithm are repeated in turn until a stopping criterion is satisfied (e.g. we could stop the iterations once the Euclidean norm of the vector $\psi^{(k+1)} - \psi^{(k)}$ falls below a threshold $\epsilon > 0$).

To initialize the algorithm, we need an initial value $\psi^{(0)}$. In [LAM 92, HAL 00], the authors choose $\beta^{(0)}$ to be the estimate of β obtained by fitting a standard Poisson model to the data. They also suggest $\hat{p}_0 := (\sum_{i=1}^n 1_{\{Z_i=0\}} - \sum_{i=1}^n \exp(-\lambda_i^{(0)}))/n$ for the initial value of the constant (or "intercept") γ_1 in γ, where $\lambda_i^{(0)}$ is obtained by substituting $\beta^{(0)}$ into equation [4.4] ($\hat{p}_0$ can be interpreted as an estimate of the zero inflation probability). Finally, [LAM 92, HAL 00] suggest a value of 0 to initialize the other components of γ.

REMARK.– As an alternative estimation approach, we can maximize the log-likelihood in equation [4.6] directly using nonlinear optimization algorithms (Newton–Raphson, etc.). This approach is, for example, implemented by the `zeroinfl` function from the `pscl` package in R (see [RCO 17, JAC 15]). In practice, the EM algorithm has proven to be a good choice for estimating the parameters of zero-inflated regression models with random effects. These models were first developed to account for correlated observations of the response variable (grouped data, longitudinal data). The indicator variables S_i and the random effects are viewed as missing variables in the EM algorithm. Interested readers can find more information in [HAL 00, HAL 04]. $\square$

4.2.2.2. *Identifiability and asymptotics*

In [ERH 06, CZA 07], the authors show that the maximum likelihood estimator $\hat{\psi}_n$ is weakly consistent and asymptotically Gaussian, i.e. as n tends to infinity, the sequence $(\hat{\psi}_n)$ converges to a Gaussian vector with mean zero and whose variance–covariance matrix is the inverse of the Fisher information matrix (which is calculated from the log-likelihood in equation [4.6]). Interested readers can refer to [ERH 06, CZA 07] for a detailed proof of these results and the full statement of the regularity conditions that are required.

The model considered by [ERH 06, CZA 07] is in fact more general than the zero-inflated Poisson model. The authors of these articles replace the Poisson distribution by a generalized Poisson distribution, which features an additional parameter modeling the dispersion (see [CON 92]). The model thus obtained (called ZIGP, for zero-inflated generalized Poisson) includes the ZIP model from equation [4.5] as a special case. The dispersion parameter can be chosen to be constant (see [CZA 05]) but can also depend on the covariables [ERH 06, CZA 07]. Any asymptotic results shown for the ZIGP model also hold in the special case of the ZIP model.

REMARK.– Establishing an interpretation of the influence of the explanatory variables can be difficult when the same variables affect both π_i and λ_i, although this does not undermine the identifiability of the model (we recall that a statistical model $(P_\theta, \theta \in \Theta)$ is said to be identifiable if the mapping $\theta \mapsto P_\theta$ is injective; intuitively, a model is said to be identifiable if distinct parameters lead to different distributions; interested readers can refer to [LI 12] for an identifiability study of the ZIP model). For this reason, many authors recommend to avoid using the same set of covariables for the vectors $\mathbf{X}_i$ and $\mathbf{W}_i$ (e.g. see [WIN 13]). $\square$

4.2.2.3. *EM algorithm: technical computations*

First, we give the full computation for the log-likelihood in equation [4.7]. With the notation from section 4.2.2.1, suppose that we are observing an independent sample $(Z_1, S_1, \mathbf{X}_1, \mathbf{W}_1)$, ..., $(Z_n, S_n, \mathbf{X}_n, \mathbf{W}_n)$. The so-called complete log-likelihood of the parameter ψ based on these observations can be computed as follows:

$$\ell_n^c(\psi) = \ln \left[\prod_{i=1}^n \mathbb{P}(Z_i = 0, S_i = 1 | \mathbf{X}_i, \mathbf{W}_i)^{S_i} \right.$$

$$\left. \times \mathbb{P}(Z_i = z_i, S_i = 0 | \mathbf{X}_i, \mathbf{W}_i)^{1-S_i} \right]$$

$$= \ln \left[\prod_{i=1}^n \{ \mathbb{P}(Z_i = 0 | S_i = 1, \mathbf{X}_i, \mathbf{W}_i) \mathbb{P}(S_i = 1 | \mathbf{X}_i, \mathbf{W}_i) \}^{S_i} \right.$$

$$\left. \times \{ \mathbb{P}(Z_i = z_i | S_i = 0, \mathbf{X}_i, \mathbf{W}_i) \mathbb{P}(S_i = 0 | \mathbf{X}_i, \mathbf{W}_i) \}^{1-S_i} \right]$$

$$= \ln \left[\prod_{i=1}^n \pi_i^{S_i} \times \left(e^{-\lambda_i} \frac{\lambda_i^{Z_i}}{Z_i!} \right)^{1-S_i} (1 - \pi_i)^{1-S_i} \right]$$

$$= \sum_{i=1}^n [S_i \ln \pi_i + (1 - S_i) \ln(1 - \pi_i) - (1 - S_i)\lambda_i + Z_i(1 - S_i) \ln \lambda_i$$

$$- (1 - S_i) \ln(Z_i!)]$$

$$= \sum_{i=1}^n \left[S_i \gamma^\top \mathbf{W}_i - \ln \left(1 + \exp \left(\gamma^\top \mathbf{W}_i \right) \right) \right]$$

$$+ \sum_{i=1}^n (1 - S_i) \left[Z_i \beta^\top \mathbf{X}_i - \exp(\beta^\top \mathbf{X}_i) - \ln(Z_i!) \right].$$

Next, we give the computation for the conditional expectation of S_i given the observations under the distribution with parameter $\psi^{(k)}$ (in the calculations below, the probability of the event A conditional on the event B under the distribution with parameter $\psi^{(k)}$ is denoted as $\mathbb{P}(A|B; \psi^{(k)})$). If $Z_i > 0$, then we necessarily have $S_i = 0$, and so $\mathbb{E}(S_i | \mathcal{O}_n; \psi^{(k)}) = \mathbb{P}(S_i = 1 | \mathcal{O}_n; \psi^{(k)}) = 0$. If $Z_i = 0$, then:

$$\mathbb{E}(S_i | \mathcal{O}_n; \psi^{(k)}) = \mathbb{P}(S_i = 1 | \mathcal{O}_n; \psi^{(k)})$$

$$= \mathbb{P}(S_i = 1 | \{ Z_i = 0 \}, \mathbf{X}_i, \mathbf{W}_i; \psi^{(k)}),$$

by the fact that the observations are independent for $i = 1, \ldots, n$. Hence:

$$
\begin{aligned}
\mathbb{E}(S_i | \mathcal{O}_n; \psi^{(k)}) &= \frac{\mathbb{P}(Z_i = 0 | S_i = 1, \mathbf{X}_i, \mathbf{W}_i; \psi^{(k)}) \cdot \mathbb{P}(S_i = 1 | \mathbf{X}_i, \mathbf{W}_i; \psi^{(k)})}{\mathbb{P}(Z_i = 0 | \mathbf{X}_i, \mathbf{W}_i; \psi^{(k)})} \\
&= \frac{\mathbb{P}(S_i = 1 | \mathbf{X}_i, \mathbf{W}_i; \psi^{(k)})}{\mathbb{P}(Z_i = 0 | \mathbf{X}_i, \mathbf{W}_i; \psi^{(k)})} \\
&= \frac{\pi_i^{(k)}}{\pi_i^{(k)} + \exp(-\lambda_i)(1 - \pi_i^{(k)})} \\
&= \left[1 + \exp\left(-\gamma^{(k)\top} \mathbf{W}_i - \exp\left(\beta^{(k)\top} \mathbf{X}_i \right) \right) \right]^{-1}.
\end{aligned}
$$

4.3. ZIB regression model

4.3.1. Definition

The zero-inflated binomial regression model was introduced by [HAL 00] to model count data with a known upper bound in the presence of zero inflation. This model has since been applied in various fields, such as entomology [VAN 00], oral and dental epidemiology [GIL 09, MAT 13], public health [HE 15] and healthcare economics [DIA 17a].

The zero-inflated binomial regression model is defined by allowing the probabilities π and p of the ZIB model to depend on the covariates. For each individual i, the model is therefore defined as:

$$
\mathbb{P}(Z_i = z) = \begin{cases} \pi_i + (1 - \pi_i)(1 - p_i)^{m_i} & z = 0 \\ (1 - \pi_i) C_{m_i}^z p_i^z (1 - p_i)^{m_i - z} & z = 1, 2, \ldots, m_i \end{cases}
$$

where π_i and p_i are functions of the covariates $\mathbf{W}_i = (W_{i1}, \ldots, W_{iq})^\top$ and $\mathbf{X}_i = (X_{i1}, \ldots, X_{ip})^\top$, respectively (setting $X_{i1} = W_{i1} = 1$). These covariables can be either qualitative or quantitative, and the vectors $\mathbf{W}_i$ and $\mathbf{X}_i$ can have shared elements (we will discuss this aspect further in section 4.3.2.2). The probabilities π_i and p_i are usually specified by logistic regressions, leading to the model:

$$\forall i = 1, \ldots, n, \quad \begin{cases} Z_i \sim \pi_i \delta_0 + (1 - \pi_i) \mathcal{B}(m_i, p_i) \\ \text{logit}(\pi_i) = \gamma^\top \mathbf{W}_i \\ \text{logit}(p_i) = \beta^\top \mathbf{X}_i \end{cases} \quad [4.8]$$

Notationally, we write that $Z_i \sim \text{ZIB}(m_i, p_i, \pi_i)$. Under this model:

$$Z_i \sim \begin{cases} 0 & \text{with probability } \pi_i \\ \mathcal{B}(m_i, p_i) & \text{with probability } 1 - \pi_i \end{cases}$$

Conditional on $\mathbf{X}_i$ and $\mathbf{W}_i$, the expected value and the variance of $Z_i \sim \text{ZIB}(m_i, p_i, \pi_i)$ are given by $\mathbb{E}(Z_i | \mathbf{X}_i, \mathbf{W}_i) = (1 - \pi_i) m_i p_i$ and $\text{var}(Z_i | \mathbf{X}_i, \mathbf{W}_i) = (1 - \pi_i) m_i p_i [1 - p_i (1 - m_i \pi_i)]$, respectively.

REMARK.– The special case where $m_i = 1$ for every i has been studied separately due to specific difficulties associated with the identifiability of the model (interested readers can refer to [DIO 11, DIO 16], as well as section 4.3.2.2 of this book). □

4.3.2. *Estimation in the ZIB model*

Let $\psi = (\beta^\top, \gamma^\top)^\top$ be the set of parameters of the model in equation [4.8]. These parameters can be estimated by the maximum likelihood method. Suppose that we have n independent observations $(Z_1, \mathbf{X}_1, \mathbf{W}_1)$, ..., $(Z_n, \mathbf{X}_n, \mathbf{W}_n)$. The likelihood is given by:

$$L_n(\psi) = \prod_{i=1}^{n} \left(\pi_i + (1 - \pi_i)(1 - p_i)^{m_i} \right)^{J_i}$$

$$\cdot \left((1 - \pi_i) C_{m_i}^{Z_i} p_i^{Z_i} (1 - p_i)^{m_i - Z_i} \right)^{1 - J_i},$$

where $J_i := 1_{\{Z_i = 0\}}$. From this, we can easily deduce the log-likelihood $\ell_n(\psi) = \ln L_n(\psi)$:

$$\ell_n(\psi) = \sum_{i=1}^{n} \left\{ J_i \ln \left(e^{\gamma^\top \mathbf{W}_i} + (1 + e^{\beta^\top \mathbf{X}_i})^{-m_i} \right) - \ln \left(1 + e^{\gamma^\top \mathbf{W}_i} \right) \right.$$

$$\left. + (1 - J_i) \left[Z_i \beta^\top \mathbf{X}_i - m_i \ln \left(1 + e^{\beta^\top \mathbf{X}_i} \right) \right] \right\},$$

which gives us the maximum likelihood estimator $\hat{\psi}_n$ of ψ after solving the following system of $p + q$ equations:

$$\frac{\partial}{\partial \psi} \ell_n(\psi) \bigg|_{\psi = \hat{\psi}_n} = 0.$$

As with the ZIP model, this estimator does not have an explicit expression. In [HAL 00], the author uses an EM-type algorithm to approximate $\hat{\psi}_n$; in [DIA 17a], the log-likelihood is maximized directly using a nonlinear optimization algorithm. The EM algorithm is described in the following section. This section can be safely skipped.

4.3.2.1. *EM algorithm*

The iterative EM algorithm approximates the maximum likelihood estimator by alternating between the E-step and the M-step. During the E-step, the conditional expectation $\mathbb{E}\left(\ell_n^c(\psi)|\mathcal{O}_n; \psi^{(k)}\right)$ of the complete log-likelihood given the observations $\mathcal{O}_n := \{(Z_1, \mathbf{X}_1, \mathbf{W}_1), \ldots, (Z_n, \mathbf{X}_n, \mathbf{W}_n)\}$ is calculated under the distribution with parameter $\psi^{(k)}$ (where $\psi^{(k)}$ denotes the estimate of ψ obtained at the k-th iteration of the algorithm). The M-step finds the value $\psi^{(k+1)} = \arg\max_\psi \mathbb{E}(\ell_n^c(\psi)|\mathcal{O}_n; \psi^{(k)})$.

As in section 4.2.2.1, let S_i be the indicator variable (unobserved in practice) that takes the value 1 if Z_i is guaranteed to be 0 and takes the value 0 if Z_i follows the binomial distribution $\mathcal{B}(m_i, p_i)$. If the S_i were observed, then the "complete" log-likelihood of ψ (i.e. the log-likelihood based on the $(Z_i, S_i, \mathbf{X}_i, \mathbf{W}_i), i = 1, \ldots, n$) would have the following expression (for details of this calculation, see section 4.3.2.4; they are similar to the calculation for the ZIP model):

$$\ell_n^c(\psi) = \sum_{i=1}^n \left[S_i \gamma^\top \mathbf{W}_i - \ln\left(1 + e^{\gamma^\top \mathbf{W}_i}\right) \right] \qquad [4.9]$$

$$+ \sum_{i=1}^n (1 - S_i) \left[Z_i \beta^\top \mathbf{X}_i - m_i \ln\left(1 + e^{\beta^\top \mathbf{X}_i}\right) + \ln C_{m_i}^{Z_i} \right].$$

The E-step of the algorithm computes the conditional expectation $\mathbb{E}\left(\ell_n^c(\psi)|\mathcal{O}_n; \psi^{(k)}\right)$, which, in this case, also reduces to computing the conditional expectation of S_i given the observations under the distribution with parameter $\psi^{(k)}$. The details of the calculation can be found in section 4.3.2.4. The conditional expectation has the expression:

$$\mathbb{E}(S_i|\mathcal{O}_n; \psi^{(k)})$$

$$= \begin{cases} 0 & \text{if } Z_i > 0 \\ \left[1 + \exp\left(-\gamma^{(k)\top}\mathbf{W}_i\right)\left(1 + \exp\left(\beta^{(k)\top}\mathbf{X}_i\right)\right)^{-m_i}\right]^{-1} & \text{if } Z_i = 0 \end{cases}$$

From this, we can deduce an expression for $\mathbb{E}\left(\ell_n^c(\psi)|\mathcal{O}_n; \psi^{(k)}\right)$:

$$\mathbb{E}\left(\ell_n^c(\psi)|\mathcal{O}_n; \psi^{(k)}\right)$$

$$= \sum_{i=1}^{n}\left[\mathbb{E}(S_i|\mathcal{O}_n; \psi^{(k)})\gamma^\top\mathbf{W}_i - \ln\left(1 + e^{\gamma^\top\mathbf{W}_i}\right)\right]$$

$$+ \sum_{i=1}^{n}(1 - \mathbb{E}(S_i|\mathcal{O}_n; \psi^{(k)}))\left[Z_i\beta^\top\mathbf{X}_i - m_i\ln\left(1 + e^{\beta^\top\mathbf{X}_i}\right) + \ln C_{m_i}^{Z_i}\right]$$

$$:= \tilde{\ell}_{n,1}(\gamma) + \tilde{\ell}_{n,2}(\beta),$$

which, like the ZIP model, splits into a sum of two terms. The first term is a function of γ only, and the second is a function of β only. The M-step can then be performed by maximizing each of these terms separately, which again reduces to the estimation of two generalized linear models, since the terms $\tilde{\ell}_{n,1}(\gamma)$ and $\tilde{\ell}_{n,2}(\beta)$ coincide with the log-likelihoods of binomial regression models.

The E- and M-steps are repeated in turn until a stopping criterion is satisfied. To initialize the algorithm, we require an initial value $\psi^{(0)}$. The estimate of β obtained by fitting a binomial regression model to the data is a reasonable choice of $\beta^{(0)}$. Similarly, the choice of $\gamma^{(0)}$ can be made according to the same principles as the ZIP model. For example, [LAM 92, HAL 00] choose $\hat{p}_0 := (\sum_{i=1}^{n} 1_{\{Z_i=0\}} - \sum_{i=1}^{n}(1 - p_i^{(0)})^{m_i})/n$ for the initial value of the constant in γ (where $p_i^{(0)}$ denotes the estimate of p_i computed using the value $\beta^{(0)}$).

REMARK.– Maximum likelihood estimation can be performed in the ZIB regression model using the `zibinomialff` and `zibinomial` functions from the VGAM package [YEE 16]. Alternatively, [DIA 17a] uses the maxLik function from the maxLik package [HEN 11]. The EM algorithm is used by [HAL 00] to estimate a ZIB regression model with random effects (which are viewed as additional missing variables by the EM algorithm alongside the indicator variables S_i).   □

4.3.2.2. *Identifiability*

The ZIB regression model is identifiable. The proof and the required regularity conditions are omitted here; they are discussed in section 4.5 for the zero-inflated multinomial (ZIM) model, which is a generalization of the ZIB model. Nevertheless, one special case deserves to be considered separately – the case where m_i is equal to 1 for all $i = 1, \ldots, n$, which can lead to a non-identifiable model. We consider the following model:

$$\forall i = 1, \ldots, n, \quad \begin{cases} Z_i \sim (1 - \pi_i)\delta_0 + \pi_i \mathcal{B}(p_i) \\ \mathrm{logit}(\pi_i) = \gamma^\top \mathbf{W}_i \\ \mathrm{logit}(p_i) = \beta^\top \mathbf{X}_i \end{cases} \quad [4.10]$$

where $\mathcal{B}(p_i) \equiv \mathcal{B}(1, p_i)$ denotes the Bernoulli distribution with parameter p_i. Suppose that we have independent observations $(Z_1, \mathbf{X}_1, \mathbf{W}_1)$, ..., $(Z_n, \mathbf{X}_n, \mathbf{W}_n)$ of this model (where each Z_i is either 0 or 1). The likelihood of (β, γ) can be computed as follows:

$$L_n(\beta, \gamma) = \prod_{i=1}^{n} \left(\mathbb{P}(Z_i = 0 | \mathbf{X}_i, \mathbf{W}_i) \right)^{1 - Z_i} \left(\mathbb{P}(Z_i = 1 | \mathbf{X}_i, \mathbf{W}_i) \right)^{Z_i}$$

$$= \prod_{i=1}^{n} \left(1 - \mathbb{P}(Z_i = 1 | \mathbf{X}_i, \mathbf{W}_i) \right)^{1 - Z_i} \left(\mathbb{P}(Z_i = 1 | \mathbf{X}_i, \mathbf{W}_i) \right)^{Z_i}$$

$$= \prod_{i=1}^{n} \left(1 - p_i \pi_i \right)^{1 - Z_i} \left(p_i \pi_i \right)^{Z_i}$$

$$= \prod_{i=1}^{n} \left(1 - \frac{e^{\beta^\top \mathbf{X}_i + \gamma^\top \mathbf{W}_i}}{(1 + e^{\beta^\top \mathbf{X}_i})(1 + e^{\gamma^\top \mathbf{W}_i})} \right)^{1 - Z_i} \quad [4.11]$$

$$\times \left(\frac{e^{\beta^\top \mathbf{X}_i + \gamma^\top \mathbf{W}_i}}{(1 + e^{\beta^\top \mathbf{X}_i})(1 + e^{\gamma^\top \mathbf{W}_i})} \right)^{Z_i}.$$

We consider now the special case, where $\mathbf{X}_i = \mathbf{W}_i$ (i.e. the same explanatory variables appear in the linear predictors of both p_i and π_i). In this case, the likelihood becomes:

$$L_n(\beta, \gamma) = \prod_{i=1}^{n} \left(1 - \frac{e^{(\beta+\gamma)^\top \mathbf{X}_i}}{(1 + e^{\beta^\top \mathbf{X}_i})(1 + e^{\gamma^\top \mathbf{X}_i})} \right)^{1-Z_i}$$
$$\times \left(\frac{e^{(\beta+\gamma)^\top \mathbf{X}_i}}{(1 + e^{\beta^\top \mathbf{X}_i})(1 + e^{\gamma^\top \mathbf{X}_i})} \right)^{Z_i}.$$

It is easy to see that $L_n(\beta, \gamma) = L_n(\gamma, \beta)$; the parameters β and γ are "interchangeable" [DIO 11], and the two distinct values (β, γ) and (γ, β) of these parameters result in the same likelihood. Hence, the model is not identifiable.

To resolve this problem, [DIO 11] suggests that the same set of explanatory variables should not be used for both p_i and π_i. In other words, the vectors $\mathbf{X}_i$ and $\mathbf{W}_i$ should differ by at least one component. However, this condition is not sufficient to guarantee identifiability for the model in equation [4.10].

To see this, we consider the following two ZIB models, which are obtained by exchanging the linear predictors of π_i and p_i:

$$\forall i = 1, \ldots, n, \quad \begin{cases} Z_i \sim (1 - \pi_i)\delta_0 + \pi_i \mathcal{B}(p_i) \\ \text{logit}(\pi_i) = \gamma^\top \mathbf{W}_i \\ \text{logit}(p_i) = \beta^\top \mathbf{X}_i \end{cases}$$

and

$$\forall i = 1, \ldots, n, \quad \begin{cases} Z_i \sim (1 - \pi_i)\delta_0 + \pi_i \mathcal{B}(p_i) \\ \text{logit}(\pi_i) = \beta^\top \mathbf{X}_i \\ \text{logit}(p_i) = \gamma^\top \mathbf{W}_i \end{cases}$$

It is easy to see that the likelihood in equation [4.11] is the same for both models (in [DIO 11], the authors use the term "interchangeability" to describe the linear predictors of p_i and π_i). It is therefore not possible to identify the models of p_i and π_i based on the observations. [DIO 11] proposes to eliminate this source of non-identifiability by requiring the following condition $\mathcal{C}$ in addition to the condition $\mathbf{X}_i \neq \mathbf{W}_i$ stated above.

$\mathcal{C}$: "There exists a continuous variable V such that, writing β_V and γ_V for the parameters associated with V in the linear predictors of p_i and π_i respectively, one of the following two conditions is satisfied: $\mathcal{C}_1 := \{\beta_V \neq 0$ and $\gamma_V = 0\}$ or $\mathcal{C}_2 := \{\beta_V = 0$ and $\gamma_V \neq 0\}$. Furthermore, it should be known a priori (i.e. at model construction) which of the two conditions $\mathcal{C}_1$ or $\mathcal{C}_2$ is satisfied."

REMARK.– If we know a priori which of the two conditions $\mathcal{C}_1$ or $\mathcal{C}_2$ is satisfied, we can unambiguously assign each of the linear predictors $\beta^\top \mathbf{X}_i$ and $\gamma^\top \mathbf{W}_i$ to the corresponding model p_i or π_i.

This condition can be viewed as an additional constraint that may be lifted under some conditions, subject to expert approval. Another solution, proposed in [DIA 17a], is to fit a logistic regression model to the observations $(1_{\{Z_1=0\}}, \mathbf{X}_1, \mathbf{W}_1), \ldots, (1_{\{Z_n=0\}}, \mathbf{X}_n, \mathbf{W}_n)$ (the response variables are given by the indicator variables $1_{\{Z_1=0\}}, \ldots, 1_{\{Z_n=0\}}$) to identify a priori any explanatory variables that do not act upon the zero-inflated model π_i. However, it should be noted that this procedure is somewhat of an approximation, since the variables $1_{\{Z_i=0\}}$ are not indicators of zero inflation (any observed zeros may be random). □

REMARK.– The continuity condition on V is a technical condition that is used in the proof of identifiability given by [DIO 11]. □

4.3.2.3. Asymptotics

In [DIA 17a], the authors show that the maximum likelihood estimator $\hat{\psi}_n$ in the ZIB model from equation [4.8] is strongly consistent (we recall that an estimator $\hat{\psi}_n$ of ψ is said to be strongly consistent if the sequence $(\hat{\psi}_n)_n$ converges almost surely (a.s.) to ψ). It is also asymptotically Gaussian. Let:

$$\ddot{\ell}_n(\psi) = \frac{\partial^2}{\partial\psi\partial\psi^\top}\ell_n(\psi)$$

be the matrix of second derivatives of $\ell_n(\psi)$, and we write $\widehat{\Sigma}_n := -\ddot{\ell}_n(\hat{\psi}_n)/n$ for the empirical Fisher information matrix. Then, as n tends to infinity, $\widehat{\Sigma}_n^{\frac{1}{2}}\sqrt{n}(\hat{\psi}_n - \psi)$ converges in distribution to a Gaussian vector of dimension $p + q$ with mean zero and whose variance–covariance matrix is the identity matrix of size $p + q$.

The regularity conditions required for this result are stated in [DIA 17a]. They are not restated here, since we will revisit them in section 4.5.4 (dedicated to the asymptotic properties of the maximum likelihood estimator in the ZIM model, which includes the ZIB model as a special case). These asymptotic results also hold in the special case where m_i is equal to 1 for all $i = 1, \ldots, n$, provided that the identifiability condition $\mathcal{C}$ holds.

4.3.2.4. *EM algorithm: technical computations*

First, we give the computation for the complete log-likelihood in equation [4.9] based on an independent sample $(Z_1, S_1, \mathbf{X}_1, \mathbf{W}_1)$, ..., $(Z_n, S_n, \mathbf{X}_n, \mathbf{W}_n)$:

$$
\ell_n^c(\psi) = \ln \left[\prod_{i=1}^n \{ \mathbb{P}(Z_i = 0 | S_i = 1, \mathbf{X}_i, \mathbf{W}_i) \mathbb{P}(S_i = 1 | \mathbf{X}_i, \mathbf{W}_i) \}^{S_i} \right.
$$

$$
\left. \times \{ \mathbb{P}(Z_i = z_i | S_i = 0, \mathbf{X}_i, \mathbf{W}_i) \mathbb{P}(S_i = 0 | \mathbf{X}_i, \mathbf{W}_i) \}^{1-S_i} \right]
$$

$$
= \ln \left[\prod_{i=1}^n \pi_i^{S_i} \times \left(C_{m_i}^{Z_i} p_i^{Z_i} (1 - p_i)^{m_i - Z_i} \right)^{1-S_i} (1 - \pi_i)^{1-S_i} \right]
$$

$$
= \sum_{i=1}^n \left[S_i \gamma^\top \mathbf{W}_i - \ln \left(1 + e^{\gamma^\top \mathbf{W}_i} \right) \right]
$$

$$
+ \sum_{i=1}^n (1 - S_i) \left[Z_i \beta^\top \mathbf{X}_i - m_i \ln \left(1 + e^{\beta^\top \mathbf{X}_i} \right) + \ln C_{m_i}^{Z_i} \right].
$$

Next, we compute the conditional expectation of S_i given the observations under the distribution with parameter $\psi^{(k)}$. If $Z_i > 0$, then we necessarily have that $S_i = 0$, and so $\mathbb{E}(S_i | \mathcal{O}_n; \psi^{(k)}) = \mathbb{P}(S_i = 1 | \mathcal{O}_n; \psi^{(k)}) = 0$. If $Z_i = 0$, then, by reasoning as in section 4.2.2.3:

$$
\mathbb{E}(S_i | \mathcal{O}_n; \psi^{(k)}) = \mathbb{P}(S_i = 1 | \{ Z_i = 0 \}, \mathbf{X}_i, \mathbf{W}_i; \psi^{(k)})
$$

$$
= \frac{\mathbb{P}(Z_i = 0 | S_i = 1, \mathbf{X}_i, \mathbf{W}_i; \psi^{(k)}) \cdot \mathbb{P}(S_i = 1 | \mathbf{X}_i, \mathbf{W}_i; \psi^{(k)})}{\mathbb{P}(Z_i = 0 | \mathbf{X}_i, \mathbf{W}_i; \psi^{(k)})}
$$

$$
= \frac{\mathbb{P}(S_i = 1|\mathbf{X}_i, \mathbf{W}_i; \psi^{(k)})}{\mathbb{P}(Z_i = 0|\mathbf{X}_i, \mathbf{W}_i; \psi^{(k)})}
$$

$$
= \frac{\pi_i^{(k)}}{\pi_i^{(k)} + (1 - p_i^{(k)})^{m_i}(1 - \pi_i^{(k)})}
$$

$$
= \left[1 + \exp\left(-\gamma^{(k)\top}\mathbf{W}_i\right)\left(1 + \exp\left(\beta^{(k)\top}\mathbf{X}_i\right)\right)^{-m_i} \right]^{-1}.
$$

4.4. Example of an application of the ZIP and ZIB models in healthcare economics

In this section, we present an illustrative application of the ZIB model (and in slightly less detail the ZIP model) to the NMES1988 data. Parts of this application are reproduced from [DIA 17a]. Interested readers can refer to [DEB 97] to find a detailed analysis performed using the ZIP model.

4.4.1. The ZIB model

The problem considered in [DIA 17a] is as follows: the goal is to identify the factors that determine how patients choose between the two types of medical appointments: i) office visits to a physician and ii) office visits to a non-physician. The authors considered individuals whose total number of office visits of both types ranged from 2 to 25.

The R code listed below plots the frequency distributions of the ofp (number of office visits to a physician) and ofnp (number of office visits to a non-physician) variables, as shown in Figures 4.8 and 4.9.

```
visits.ofp=factor(ofp, levels=0:max(ofp))
visits.tab=table(visits.ofp)
barplot(visits.tab, xlab="Number of office visits to a
    physician", ylab="Frequency",col="lightblue")

visits.ofnp=factor(ofnp, levels=0:max(ofnp))
visits.tab=table(visits.ofnp)
barplot(visits.tab, xlab="Number of office visits to a
    non-physician", ylab="Frequency",col="lightblue")
```

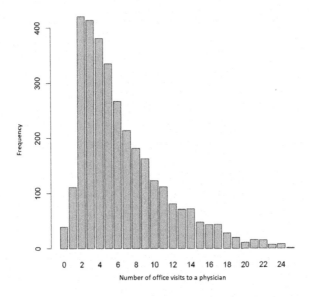

Figure 4.8. *Frequency distribution of the number of office visits to a physician*

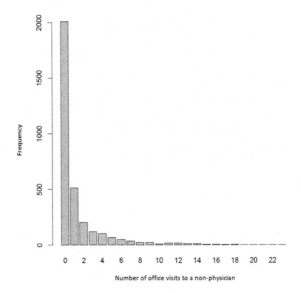

Figure 4.9. *Frequency distribution of the number of office visits to a non-physician*

The proportions of zeros in the observations of ofp and ofnp are given by 0.0121 and 0.6219, respectively. Figure 4.9, together with the high proportion of zeros observed for the ofnp variable, suggest that we are faced with a zero-inflated problem.

For each individual i ($i = 1, \ldots, n = 3227$) in the sample, let Z_i be the number of office visits to a non-physician and let m_i be the total number of office visits (either to a physician or a non-physician). We shall model the variable Z_i given m_i with a ZIB model:

$$Z_i \sim \pi_i \delta_0 + (1 - \pi_i) \mathcal{B}(m_i, p_i),$$

where:

$- \pi_i$ is the probability that the i-th patient systematically avoids all office visits to a non-physician,

$- p_i$ is the probability that a patient who is prepared to visit a non-physician does indeed request an appointment.

The analysis considers the following explanatory variables:

– gender (coded as 1 for women, 0 for men): gender,

– age (in years /10): age,

– marital status (coded as 1 if the patient is married, 0 otherwise): fstatus,

– duration of education (in years): school,

– household income of the patient (in tens of thousands of US dollars): income,

– number of chronic diseases (cancer, diabetes, etc.) suffered by the patient: numchron,

– a variable indicating whether the patient is covered by Medicaid (health insurance provided to low-income families and individuals), coded as 1 if the patient is covered, 0 otherwise: med,

– a variable indicating the patient's self-perception of his or her state of health (excellent, average, poor): health.

We shall recode the health variable in terms of two indicator variables: health1, which takes the value 1 if the patient perceives his or her own health to be poor and 0 otherwise, and health2, which takes the value 1 if the patient perceives his or her own health to be excellent and 0 otherwise.

We shall begin by estimating a ZIB model in which all available explanatory variables are included in the linear predictors of p_i and π_i. This model may be stated as follows:

$$
\begin{cases}
Z_i \sim \pi_i \delta_0 + (1 - \pi_i)\mathcal{B}(m_i, p_i) \\[2mm]
\begin{aligned}
\text{logit}(p_i) &= \beta_1 + \beta_2\,\text{health1}_i + \beta_3\,\text{health2}_i + \beta_4\,\text{numchron}_i + \beta_5\,\text{age}_i \\
&\quad + \beta_6\,\text{gender}_i + \beta_7\,\text{fstatus}_i + \beta_8\,\text{school}_i + \beta_9\,\text{income}_i + \beta_{10}\,\text{med}_i
\end{aligned} \\[2mm]
\begin{aligned}
\text{logit}(\pi_i) &= \gamma_1 + \gamma_2\,\text{health1}_i + \gamma_3\,\text{health2}_i + \gamma_4\,\text{numchron}_i + \gamma_5\,\text{age}_i \\
&\quad + \gamma_6\,\text{gender}_i + \gamma_7\,\text{fstatus}_i + \gamma_8\,\text{school}_i + \gamma_9\,\text{income}_i + \gamma_{10}\,\text{med}_i
\end{aligned}
\end{cases}
$$

where health1_i, health2_i, numchron_i, etc., denote the values taken by the variables health1, health2, numchron, etc., respectively, on the i-th individual. We shall maximize the log-likelihood using the Newton–Raphson algorithm, which is implemented by the maxLik function from the maxLik package [HEN 11]. This function returns the following output:

```
Maximum Likelihood estimation
Newton-Raphson maximisation, 7 iterations
Return code 2: successive function values within
      tolerance limit
Log-Likelihood: -9434.112
20   free parameters
Estimates:
          Estimate  Std. error  t value   Pr(> t)
  [1,]  -0.246865    0.324306   -0.761  0.446532
  [2,]  -0.347136    0.075012   -4.628  3.70e-06  ***
  [3,]   0.271371    0.083836    3.237  0.001208  **
  [4,]  -0.092138    0.016976   -5.428  5.71e-08  ***
  [5,]  -0.051720    0.039240   -1.318  0.187493
  [6,]   0.067600    0.048933    1.381  0.167129
  [7,]   0.133499    0.048772    2.737  0.006197  **
  [8,]  -0.002979    0.006771   -0.440  0.659933
  [9,]  -0.007123    0.006471   -1.101  0.270966
  [10,]  -0.093732    0.094018   -0.997  0.318782
  [11,]   0.771511    0.768375    1.004  0.315340
```

```
[12,]   0.312812    0.137748    2.271 0.023153 *
[13,]   0.064855    0.167582    0.387 0.698751
[14,]   0.017234    0.033668    0.512 0.608745
[15,]   0.044969    0.093694    0.480 0.631262
[16,]  -0.340106    0.096232   -3.534 0.000409 ***
[17,]  -0.041497    0.100779   -0.412 0.680512
[18,]  -0.072999    0.013288   -5.494 3.94e-08 ***
[19,]  -0.002153    0.015360   -0.140 0.888534
[20,]   0.431404    0.164074    2.629 0.008555 **
---
Signif. codes: 0 '***' 0.001'**' 0.01'*' 0.05'.' 0.1 '' 1
```

REMARK.– The coefficients [1,] to [10,] (respectively, [11,] to [20,]) correspond to the parameters β_1 to β_{10} (respectively, γ_1 to γ_{10}). The estimates of these parameters are listed in the "Estimate" column. The "Std. error" column (short for "standard error") lists the estimates of the asymptotic standard deviations of each estimator. The Wald statistic for the test problems:

$$H_0 : \beta_j = 0 \quad \text{against} \quad H_1 : \beta_j \neq 0, \quad \text{for } j = 1, \ldots, 10,$$

and

$$H_0 : \gamma_j = 0 \quad \text{against} \quad H_1 : \gamma_j \neq 0, \quad \text{for } j = 1, \ldots, 10,$$

is listed in the "t value" column. This statistic is calculated as the ratio "Estimate / Std. error"; under the corresponding null hypothesis, it is asymptotically distributed like the Gaussian distribution $\mathcal{N}(0, 1)$. Thus, the absolute value of the entries in the "t value" column should be compared with the quantile of order $1 - \alpha/2$ of the distribution $\mathcal{N}(0, 1)$, where α denotes the level of the test (often chosen as $\alpha = 0.05$, in which case the corresponding quantile is approximately 1.96). Here, R instead lists the "p-value" (denoted "Pr($>$t)"), which is defined as the probability for which the distribution $\mathcal{N}(0, 1)$ (and more generally the distribution of the test statistic under H_0) takes a value greater than or equal to the observed test statistic. We reject H_0 whenever the p-value is smaller than the level α of the test.   □

The next step is to perform automatic selection of variables based on the Akaike information criterion. This leads us to retain the following ZIB model:

$$
\begin{cases}
Z_i \sim \pi_i \delta_0 + (1 - \pi_i)\mathcal{B}(m_i, p_i) \\[2mm]
\text{logit}(p_i) = \beta_1 + \beta_2\,\text{health1}_i + \beta_3\,\text{health2}_i + \beta_4\,\text{numchron}_i + \beta_5\,\text{age}_i \\
\qquad\qquad + \beta_6\,\text{gender}_i + \beta_7\,\text{fstatus}_i \\[2mm]
\text{logit}(\pi_i) = \gamma_1 + \gamma_2\,\text{health1}_i + \gamma_3\,\text{gender}_i + \gamma_4\,\text{school}_i + \gamma_5\,\text{med}_i
\end{cases}
$$

The estimates of the γ_j and the β_j are listed in Table 4.1, which also gives the corresponding standard errors, Wald statistics and p-values.

parameter	variable	estimate	s.e.	Wald test	Pr(>t)	
β_1	constant	-0.27175	0.30115	-0.902	0.366866	
β_2	health1	-0.34707	0.07387	-4.699	2.62e-06	***
β_3	health2	0.24778	0.08116	3.053	0.002265	**
β_4	numchron	-0.09491	0.01662	-5.709	1.14e-08	***
β_5	age	-0.05560	0.03868	-1.437	0.150645	
β_6	gender	0.07005	0.04857	1.442	0.149213	
β_7	fstatus	0.13250	0.04681	2.831	0.004644	**
γ_1	constant	1.09045	0.15373	7.093	1.31e-12	***
γ_2	health1	0.33179	0.13332	2.489	0.012819	*
γ_3	gender	-0.32271	0.08737	-3.694	0.000221	***
γ_4	school	-0.07299	0.01220	-5.982	2.20e-09	***
γ_5	med	0.48146	0.15969	3.015	0.002569	**

Table 4.1. *Estimate of the ZIB model based on the NMES data*

Analyzing the results in Table 4.1 gives the following insight. The variables retained in the zero-inflated model π_i are health1, gender, school and med. The probability that a patient who has decided to visit a healthcare practitioner systematically chooses a physician (and therefore systematically avoids non-physicians) is higher in patients who judge their state of health to be poor (one reasonable interpretation is that a degrading state of health prompts patients to prefer more medically oriented appointments). This probability is also higher in Medicaid beneficiaries. This is not surprising, since Medicaid coverage primarily consists of medical care[1]. The probability that a patient avoids visiting non-physicians decreases with the duration of his or her education. An analogous observation was reported by [DEB 97]. The authors suggest that higher levels of education may be associated with higher awareness of the range of healthcare services available, leading better-educated patients to diversify their healthcare consumption.

The significant explanatory variables (to the 5% level) retained in the binomial part of the ZIB model are health1, health2, numchron and fstatus. The probability of a patient visiting a non-physician decreases if the patient perceives his or her health (evaluated through the health1, health2 and numchron variables) to be poor. Intuitively, this observation seems reasonable, since we can expect patients in poor health to prioritize more medically oriented appointments with physicians. The probability of seeking an appointment with a non-physician is higher among patients who are married. One possible explanation is that married patients, who tend to be more comfortable financially, are more likely to diversify their healthcare consumption.

REMARK.– The zibinomialff and zibinomial functions from the VGAM package [YEE 16] can be used to estimate special cases of the model in equation [4.8]. The zibinomialff function estimates a ZIB model in which the zero inflation probabilities $\pi_i, i = 1, \ldots, n$ are all equal. The following R code:

```
fit=vglm(cbind(ofnp,mi-ofnp)~health1+health2+numchron+age
    +gender+fstatus+school+income+med,zibinomialff)
summary(fit)
```

---

1 Federal law in the US requires each state to include a certain number of services in their Medicaid coverage (such as hospitalization fees, hospital outpatient appointments, dental care for children, etc.) but allows each state to choose whether to expand this coverage to other types of service (dental care for adults, speech therapy, ergotherapy, etc.). Source: https://www.medicaid.gov/.

estimates the model:

$$\begin{cases} Z_i \sim \pi_i \delta_0 + (1 - \pi_i)\mathcal{B}(m_i, p_i) \\[2mm] \text{logit}(\pi_i) = \gamma \\[2mm] \text{logit}(p_i) = \beta_1 + \beta_2\,\text{health1}_i + \beta_3\,\text{health2}_i + \beta_4\,\text{numchron}_i + \beta_5\,\text{age}_i \\ \qquad\quad + \beta_6\,\text{gender}_i + \beta_7\,\text{fstatus}_i + \beta_8\,\text{school}_i + \beta_9\,\text{income}_i + \beta_{10}\,\text{med}_i \end{cases}$$

returning the output:

```
Coefficients:
                 Estimate  Std. Error  z value  Pr(>|z|)
(Intercept):1   -0.319196    0.309061   -1.033   0.30170
(Intercept):2   -0.188268    0.040785   -4.616  3.91e-06  ***
health1         -0.387716    0.070004   -5.539  3.05e-08  ***
health2          0.272340    0.093353    2.917   0.00353   **
numchron        -0.094448    0.017252   -5.475  4.38e-08  ***
age             -0.056551    0.037881   -1.493   0.13547
gender           0.100632    0.050623    1.988   0.04683   *
fstatus          0.141082    0.051886    2.719   0.00655   **
school           0.004949    0.006649    0.744   0.45672
income          -0.007408    0.007711   -0.961   0.33672
med             -0.161865    0.084938   -1.906   0.05669   .
---
Signif. codes:  0 '***' 0.001 '**' 0.01 '*' 0.05 '.' 0.1 ' ' 1
```

where the coefficients (Intercept):1 and (Intercept):2 correspond to β_1 and $-\gamma$. The parameterization used by zibinomialff is as follows: $\text{logit}(1 - \pi_i) = $ (Intercept):2, giving $\pi_i = \exp(-(\text{Intercept}):2)/(1 + \exp(-(\text{Intercept}):2))$.

The zibinomial function estimates a ZIB model in which the linear predictors $\beta^\top \mathbf{X}_i$ and $\gamma^\top \mathbf{W}_i$ share the same set of explanatory variables, i.e. $\mathbf{X}_i = \mathbf{W}_i$. The code:

```
fit=vglm(cbind(ofnp,mi-ofnp)~health1+health2+numchron+age
    +gender+fstatus+school+income+med,zibinomial)
summary(fit)
```

estimates the model:

$$
\begin{cases}
Z_i \sim \pi_i \delta_0 + (1 - \pi_i)\mathcal{B}(m_i, p_i) \\[2mm]
\text{logit}(\pi_i) = \gamma_1 + \gamma_2\,\text{health1}_i + \gamma_3\,\text{health2}_i + \gamma_4\,\text{numchron}_i + \gamma_5\,\text{age}_i \\
\qquad\qquad + \gamma_6\,\text{gender}_i + \gamma_7\,\text{fstatus}_i + \gamma_8\,\text{school}_i + \gamma_9\,\text{income}_i + \gamma_{10}\,\text{med}_i \\[2mm]
\text{logit}(p_i) = \beta_1 + \beta_2\,\text{health1}_i + \beta_3\,\text{health2}_i + \beta_4\,\text{numchron}_i + \beta_5\,\text{age}_i \\
\qquad\qquad + \beta_6\,\text{gender}_i + \beta_7\,\text{fstatus}_i + \beta_8\,\text{school}_i + \beta_9\,\text{income}_i + \beta_{10}\,\text{med}_i
\end{cases}
$$

and returns the results:

```
Coefficients:
                 Estimate Std. Error  z value Pr(>|z|)
(Intercept):1    0.771925   0.578727    1.334 0.182259
(Intercept):2   -0.246577   0.318698   -0.774 0.439108
health1:1        0.312736   0.135609    2.306 0.021102 *
health1:2       -0.347139   0.078044   -4.448 8.67e-06 ***
health2:1        0.064870   0.165714    0.391 0.695459
health2:2        0.271331   0.091892    2.953 0.003150 **
numchron:1       0.017237   0.032961    0.523 0.601010
numchron:2      -0.092139   0.017718   -5.200 1.99e-07 ***
age:1            0.044923   0.071032    0.632 0.527106
age:2           -0.051753   0.039123   -1.323 0.185891
gender:1        -0.340154   0.094588   -3.596 0.000323 ***
gender:2         0.067584   0.051885    1.303 0.192720
fstatus:1       -0.041551   0.097932   -0.424 0.671359
fstatus:2        0.133468   0.052030    2.565 0.010312 *
school:1        -0.073000   0.012756   -5.723 1.05e-08 ***
school:2        -0.002980   0.006991   -0.426 0.669891
income:1        -0.002153   0.015121   -0.142 0.886792
income:2        -0.007122   0.007399   -0.963 0.335745
med:1            0.431491   0.163598    2.638 0.008352 **
med:2           -0.093761   0.099603   -0.941 0.346529
---
Signif. codes:  0 '***' 0.001'**' 0.01'*' 0.05'.' 0.1 ' ' 1
```

In this table, the estimates associated with the variables marked with a 1 (e.g. health1:1 and numchron:1) correspond to the γ_j. The estimates associated with the variables marked 2 (e.g. health1:2 and numchron:2) correspond to the β_j. The zibinomialff and zibinomial functions use the Fisher-scoring algorithm to maximize the likelihood. $\qquad\square$

4.4.2. *ZIP model*

Let us now apply the ZIP model to the NMES1988 data set. The goal of this section is simply to present the tools for estimating ZIP regression models in R. Readers interested in a more in-depth analysis of the data can refer to [DEB 97].

Figure 4.10 shows the frequency distribution of the ofnp variable (number of office visits to a non-physician). The proportion of zeros in the observations of this variable is equal to 0.6818. This is extremely high, which together with Figure 4.10 suggests that we are in the presence of zero inflation.

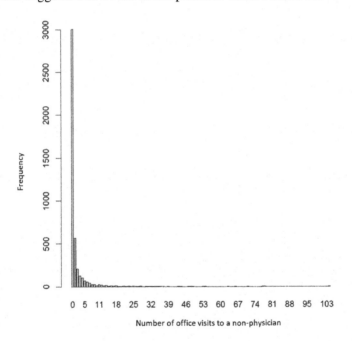

Figure 4.10. *Frequency distribution of the number of office visits to a non-physician*

For each individual i $(i = 1, \ldots, n = 4406)$ in the sample, let Z_i be the number of office visits to a non-physician. A ZIP model for Z_i may be stated as follows:

$$Z_i \sim \pi_i \delta_0 + (1 - \pi_i)\mathcal{P}(\lambda_i),$$

where:

$-\pi_i$ is the probability that the i-th patient systematically avoids visiting non-physicians,

$-\lambda_i$ is the mean number of office visits to a non-physician whenever the i-th patient is prepared to seek such a visit.

We consider again the explanatory variables health1, health2, numchron, age, gender, fstatus, school, income and med, and let us estimate the following ZIP model (called the "ZIP1 model" below):

$$
\begin{cases}
Z_i \sim \pi_i \delta_0 + (1 - \pi_i)\mathcal{P}(\lambda_i) \\[2mm]
\begin{aligned}
\text{logit}(\pi_i) = {} & \gamma_1 + \gamma_2 \, \text{health1}_i + \gamma_3 \, \text{health2}_i + \gamma_4 \, \text{numchron}_i + \gamma_5 \, \text{age}_i \\
& + \gamma_6 \, \text{gender}_i + \gamma_7 \, \text{fstatus}_i + \gamma_8 \, \text{school}_i + \gamma_9 \, \text{income}_i + \gamma_{10} \, \text{med}_i
\end{aligned} \\[2mm]
\begin{aligned}
\ln(\lambda_i) = {} & \beta_1 + \beta_2 \, \text{health1}_i + \beta_3 \, \text{health2}_i + \beta_4 \, \text{numchron}_i + \beta_5 \, \text{age}_i \\
& + \beta_6 \, \text{gender}_i + \beta_7 \, \text{fstatus}_i + \beta_8 \, \text{school}_i + \beta_9 \, \text{income}_i + \beta_{10} \, \text{med}_i
\end{aligned}
\end{cases}
$$

The zeroinfl function from the pscl package [JAC 15] provides maximum likelihood estimates of the γ_j and the β_j (obtained using nonlinear optimization algorithms). The syntax of this function is as follows:

```
zeroinfl(ofnp~health1+health2+numchron+age+gender+fstatus
    +school+income+med|health1+health2+numchron+age+gender
    +fstatus+school+income+med,dist="poisson")
```

The linear predictors of λ_i and π_i are defined in this order, separated by the pipe symbol |. If the same explanatory variables are used for both linear predictors, the syntax can be simplified:

```
ZIP1=zeroinfl(ofnp~health1+health2+numchron+age+gender+
    fstatus+school+income+med,dist="poisson")
```

The above lines of code produce the following output in R:

```
Count model coefficients (poisson with log link):
            Estimate Std. Error z value Pr(>|z|)
(Intercept)  2.590005   0.176355  14.686  < 2e-16 ***
```

```
health1        -0.003330    0.042022    -0.079  0.936846
health2         0.078577    0.046472     1.691  0.090869  .
numchron        0.042027    0.009564     4.394  1.11e-05  ***
age            -0.169648    0.021946    -7.730  1.07e-14  ***
gender         -0.049673    0.027693    -1.794  0.072858  .
fstatus        -0.005969    0.028282    -0.211  0.832852
school          0.023503    0.003912     6.007  1.89e-09  ***
income         -0.016585    0.004568    -3.631  0.000283  ***
med             0.198576    0.050466     3.935  8.33e-05  ***

Zero-inflation model coefficients (binomial with logit
     link):
                 Estimate Std. Error  z value  Pr(>|z|)
(Intercept)      1.734052    0.450189     3.852  0.000117  ***
health1          0.282331    0.111995     2.521  0.011705  *
health2          0.199730    0.129022     1.548  0.121616
numchron        -0.126513    0.026124    -4.843  1.28e-06  ***
age              0.045334    0.055898     0.811  0.417361
gender          -0.387869    0.074373    -5.215  1.84e-07  ***
fstatus         -0.083249    0.077051    -1.080  0.279950
school          -0.085720    0.010127    -8.465  < 2e-16   ***
income          -0.004365    0.011927    -0.366  0.714422
med              0.320088    0.133817     2.392  0.016758  *
---
Signif. codes: 0 '***' 0.001 '**' 0.01 '*' 0.05 '.' 0.1 ' ' 1

Log-likelihood: -9767 on 20 Df
```

The `zeroinfl` function allows us to use different explanatory variables in the linear predictors of λ_i and π_i. For example, the line of code:

```
ZIP2=zeroinfl(ofnp~health1+health2+numchron+age+gender+
      fstatus+school+income+med|numchron+age+gender+fstatus+
      school+income+med,dist="poisson")
```

estimates the following ZIP model (called the "ZIP2 model" below):

$$
\begin{cases}
Z_i \sim \pi_i \delta_0 + (1 - \pi_i)\mathcal{P}(\lambda_i) \\[2mm]
\text{logit}(\pi_i) = \gamma_1^* + \gamma_2^* \text{ numchron}_i + \gamma_3^* \text{ age}_i + \gamma_4^* \text{ gender}_i + \gamma_5^* \text{ fstatus}_i \\
\qquad\qquad + \gamma_6^* \text{ school}_i + \gamma_7^* \text{ income}_i + \gamma_8^* \text{ med}_i \\[2mm]
\ln(\lambda_i) = \beta_1^* + \beta_2^* \text{ health1}_i + \beta_3^* \text{ health2}_i + \beta_4^* \text{ numchron}_i + \beta_5^* \text{ age}_i \\
\qquad\qquad + \beta_6^* \text{ gender}_i + \beta_7^* \text{ fstatus}_i + \beta_8^* \text{ school}_i + \beta_9^* \text{ income}_i + \beta_{10}^* \text{ med}_i
\end{cases}
$$

The output produced by `zeroinfl` is as follows:

```
Count model coefficients (poisson with log link):
            Estimate Std. Error z value Pr(>|z|)
(Intercept)  2.590907   0.176376  14.690  < 2e-16  ***
health1     -0.005840   0.042161  -0.139 0.889823
health2      0.077278   0.046568   1.659 0.097023  .
numchron     0.042167   0.009563   4.409 1.04e-05 ***
age         -0.169741   0.021949  -7.733 1.05e-14 ***
gender      -0.049753   0.027693  -1.797 0.072399  .
fstatus     -0.005944   0.028282  -0.210 0.833525
school       0.023491   0.003912   6.004 1.92e-09 ***
income      -0.016568   0.004564  -3.630 0.000284 ***
med          0.199257   0.050469   3.948 7.88e-05 ***

Zero-inflation model coefficients (binomial with logit
    link):
            Estimate Std. Error z value Pr(>|z|)
(Intercept)  1.735860   0.448748   3.868  0.00011 ***
numchron    -0.111468   0.024465  -4.556 5.21e-06 ***
age          0.050115   0.055705   0.900  0.36830
gender      -0.389089   0.074249  -5.240 1.60e-07 ***
fstatus     -0.083512   0.076891  -1.086  0.27744
school      -0.087007   0.010052  -8.655  < 2e-16 ***
income      -0.004196   0.011876  -0.353  0.72388
med          0.346807   0.133280   2.602  0.00927 **
---
Signif. codes: 0 '***' 0.001'**' 0.01'*' 0.05'.' 0.1'' 1

Log-likelihood: -9771 on 18 Df
```

We can now test $H_0 : \gamma_2 = \gamma_3 = 0$ against $H_1 : (\gamma_2 \neq 0 \text{ or } \gamma_3 \neq 0)$ in the ZIP1 model, which is equivalent to testing the significance of the `health` variable (recoded as `health1` and `health2`) in the linear predictor of π_i by comparing the nested models ZIP1 and ZIP2 using a likelihood-ratio test. This test is implemented by the `lrtest` function from the `lmtest` package [ZEI 02]. Its syntax is as follows:

```
lrtest(ZIP2,ZIP1)
```

This gives the following output:

```
Likelihood ratio test

Model 1: ofnp ~ health1 + health2 + numchron + age +
    gender + fstatus +  school + income + med | numchron +
    age + gender + fstatus + school + income + med
Model 2: ofnp ~ health1 + health2 + numchron + age +
    gender + fstatus + school + income + med | health1 +
    health2 + numchron + age +  gender + fstatus + school
    + income + med
  #Df  LogLik Df  Chisq Pr(>Chisq)
1  18 -9771.3
2  20 -9767.0  2 8.6395     0.0133 *
---
Signif. codes: 0 '***' 0.001'**' 0.01'*' 0.05'.' 0.1 '' 1
```

Finally, we can perform automatic selection of variables in the ZIP regression model using the stepAIC function from the MASS package [VEN 02]. The line of code:

```
stepAIC(ZIP1)
```

returns the output:

```
Start:   AIC=19573.97
ofnp ~ health1 + health2 + numchron + age + gender +
    fstatus + school + income + med

             Df   AIC
- fstatus    2 19571
<none>         19574
- health2    2 19575
- health1    2 19577
- income     2 19585
- med        2 19590
- gender     2 19600
- numchron   2 19613
- age        2 19633
- school     2 19684

Step:   AIC=19571.18
ofnp ~ health1 + health2 + numchron + age + gender +
    school + income + med
```

```
            Df   AIC
<none>           19571
- health2    2   19572
- health1    2   19574
- income     2   19583
- med        2   19589
- gender     2   19597
- numchron   2   19611
- age        2   19632
- school     2   19682
```

4.5. ZIM regression model

The ZIP and ZIB models allow us to model univariate count data in the presence of zero inflation. However, many applications involve multivariate counts with interdependent components. This section describes a zero-inflated regression model developed by [DIA 18] to handle this type of situation.

4.5.1. *An introductory example*

Healthcare consumption and renunciation provide an example of a situation in which multiple interdependent counts are observed. In modern healthcare systems, patients typically have access to a wide range of healthcare services, for example, including the option of visiting a physician either in an office setting or at the hospital and visiting a non-physician either in an office setting or at the hospital. The ZIP and ZIB models can only consider a single measure of healthcare consumption at once and are therefore unsuitable for situations involving a multivariate response. They can of course be used to model each of the various observed counts separately, but it is usually reasonable to expect that measures of the consumption of different types of healthcare will be mutually dependent.

For example, [GUR 00] and [WAN 03] analyzed a survey performed in Australia in 1977–1978 on the healthcare consumption of 5,190 patients. Several measures of this consumption were recorded, including Z_1, the number of visits to a physician, and Z_2, the number of visits to a non-physician. In [GUR 00], the authors show that these two measures are not independent. Furthermore, these quantities are both subject to zero inflation:

the proportion of zeros observed for Z_1 (respectively Z_2) is 0.80 (respectively 0.91). However, this zero inflation also affects the pair (Z_1, Z_2) directly. The proportion of observations of the form $(Z_1, Z_2) = (0, 0)$ in the data is equal to 0.737. This means that almost three quarters of the patients never sought the healthcare services associated with either Z_1 or Z_2 (over the duration of the study). In this example, zero inflation affects the variables Z_1 and Z_2 jointly.

Several models have been proposed for zero-inflated multivariate count data: multivariate Poisson models [LI 99, LIU 15, YAN 16, FAR 17a, WAN 17], as well as bivariate negative binomial models [WAN 03, FAR 17b]. Here, we shall describe the zero-inflated regression model proposed by [DIA 18] for a multivariate count that follows a multinomial distribution. The NMES1988 data will be used to illustrate this model.

To simplify the notation, we shall only consider three measures of healthcare consumption, but the model described below is easy to generalize to J measures. These three measures are: i) the number Z_1 of office visits to a non-physician; ii) the number Z_2 of outpatient appointments[2] with a non-physician and iii) the number Z_3 of office visits to a physician. In the R codes listed below, the variable names of each of the counts Z_1, Z_2 and Z_3 are given by ofnp, opnp and ofp, respectively.

In [DIA 18], the authors consider the subset of individuals whose total number of office visits of any of these three types ranged from 2 to 25. The frequency distributions of the variables Z_1, Z_2, Z_3 on this subsample (of size 3,224) are shown in Figures 4.11, 4.12 and 4.13. The code listed below was used to generate Figure 4.11 and can easily be adapted to obtain the two other figures.

```
visits.ofnp=factor(ofnp, levels=0:max(ofnp))
visits.tab=table(visits.ofnp)
barplot(visits.tab, xlab="Number of office visits to a
    non-physician", ylab="Frequency",col="lightblue")
```

---

2 Recall that an outpatient or ambulatory appointment is conducted by hospital practitioners but does not involve hospitalization.

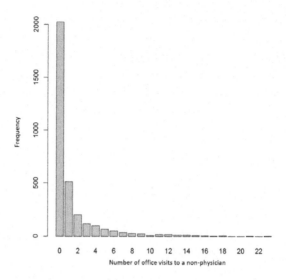

Figure 4.11. *Frequency distribution of the number of office visits to a non-physician*

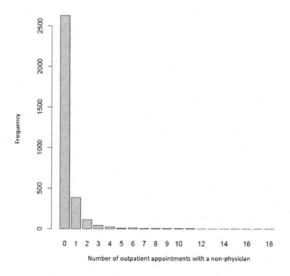

Figure 4.12. *Frequency distribution of the number of outpatient appointments with a non-physician*

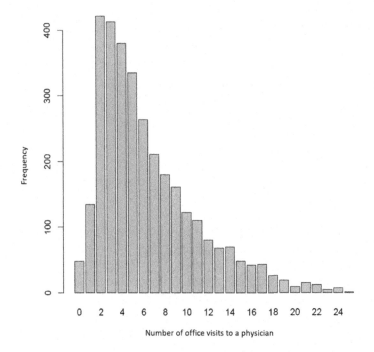

Figure 4.13. *Frequency distribution of the number of office visits to a physician*

Table 4.2 lists the proportion of zeros observed for each of the three variables.

variable	Z_1 (ofnp)	Z_2 (opnp)	Z_3 (ofp)
proportion of zeros	0.6272	0.8136	0.0149

Table 4.2. *Proportion of zeros observed for Z_1, Z_2, Z_3*

The high proportions of zeros listed in Table 4.2 for the variables Z_1 and Z_2, together with Figures 4.11 and 4.12, suggest that we are in the presence of zero inflation. Table 4.3 gives the proportion of observations of the form $(0, 0)$ for each of the three pairs of variables (Z_1, Z_2), (Z_1, Z_3) and (Z_2, Z_3).

couple (Z_i, Z_j)	(Z_1, Z_2) (ofnp, opnp)	(Z_1, Z_3) (ofnp, ofp)	(Z_2, Z_3) (opnp, ofp)
proportion of $(0, 0)$	0.5171	0.0025	0.0105

Table 4.3. *Proportion of $(0, 0)$ observed for $(Z_1, Z_2), (Z_1, Z_3), (Z_2, Z_3)$*

This table suggests that a high proportion of patients choose to never visit a non-physician, whether in an office or an outpatient setting. The frequency distribution of the pair (Z_1, Z_2) is represented graphically in Figure 4.14, which was created using the hist3D function from the plot3D package [SOE 16]:

```
hist3D(z=table(ofnp,opnp),border="black",theta=55,phi=15)
```

The frequency distribution is shown from two different angles to give a better impression of its shape.

Together, these results suggest that zero inflation is not only present in the variables Z_1 and Z_2 but also in the pair (Z_1, Z_2).

For this type of situation, which features a multivariate count with bounded components where the zero inflation affects multiple components simultaneously, [DIA 18] proposes a new zero-inflated model called the zero-inflated multinomial (ZIM) regression model. The following section gives a definition of this model.

4.5.2. *Definition of the model and estimation*

First, we recall the definition of the multinomial distribution: we say that a random variable $Z = (Z_1, \ldots, Z_r)$ of size $r \geq 2$ follows a multinomial distribution with parameters $m \in \mathbb{N} \backslash \{0\}$ and $\mathbf{p} = (p_1, p_2, \ldots, p_r) \in]0, 1[^r$, where $p_1 + p_2 + \ldots + p_r = 1$, if, for all $(z_1, \ldots, z_r) \in \{0, 1, \ldots, m\}^r$:

$$\mathbb{P}(Z = (z_1, z_2 \ldots, z_r)) = \begin{cases} \frac{m!}{z_1! z_2! \ldots z_r!} p_1^{z_1} p_2^{z_2} \cdots p_r^{z_r} & \text{if } z_1 + z_2 + \ldots + z_r = m \\ 0 & \text{otherwise} \end{cases}$$

Notationally, we write that $Z \sim \text{mult}(m, \mathbf{p})$.

Returning to the NMES1988 data, let m_i (for $i = 1, \ldots, n$) be the total number of times that the i-th patient sought healthcare of type ofnp, opnp or ofp over the duration of the study. Suppose that we wish to model the number $Z_i := (Z_{1i}, Z_{2i}, Z_{3i})$ of these visits by a multinomial distribution. To account for the inflated number of observations of type $Z_i = (0, 0, m_i)$ demonstrated in section 4.5.1 (see Table 4.3 and Figure 4.14), [DIA 18] proposes the following model:

$$Z_i \sim \begin{cases} (0, 0, m_i) & \text{with probability } \pi \\ \text{mult}(m_i, \mathbf{p}_i) & \text{with probability } 1 - \pi \end{cases} \qquad [4.12]$$

where $\mathbf{p} = (p_{1i}, p_{2i}, p_{3i})$ satisfies $p_{ji} \in]0, 1[$, $j = 1, 2, 3$, and $p_{1i} + p_{2i} + p_{3i} = 1$ (these probability values may depend on i via the explanatory variables $\mathbf{X}_i$).

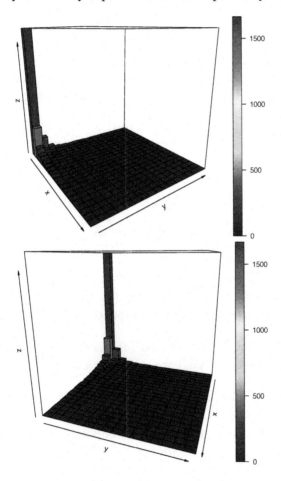

Figure 4.14. *Two representations of the frequency distribution of the pair (Z_1, Z_2) (from two different viewing angles). For a color version of the figure, please see www.iste.co.uk/dupuy/countdata.zip*

The quantity p_{1i} denotes the probability that the i-th patient chooses to visit a non-physician in an office setting (i.e. seeks healthcare of type ofnp) given that he or she can choose among ofnp, opnp and ofp and has not systematically renounced all healthcare of types ofnp and opnp. The probabilities p_{2i} and p_{3i} can be interpreted similarly.

Finally, π is the probability that a patient systematically avoids visiting any non-physician, whether in an office or outpatient setting. This is therefore the inflation probability associated with observations of type $(Z_1, Z_2) = (0, 0)$ (in this case, $Z_{3,i} = m_i$).

Let S_i be the indicator variable (unobserved in practice) that takes the value 1 if Z_i is guaranteed to be $(0, 0, m_i)$ and 0 if Z_i follows the distribution $\text{mult}(m_i, \mathbf{p}_i)$. Under the model from equation [4.12], we have:

$$\mathbb{P}(Z_i = (0, 0, m_i)|\mathbf{X}_i) = \underbrace{\mathbb{P}(Z_i = (0, 0, m_i)|\mathbf{X}_i, S_i = 1)}_{=1} \cdot \pi$$

$$+ \mathbb{P}(Z_i = (0, 0, m_i)|\mathbf{X}_i, S_i = 0) \cdot (1 - \pi)$$

$$= \pi \cdot (1 - \mathbb{P}(\text{mult}(m_i, \mathbf{p}_i) = (0, 0, m_i)|\mathbf{X}_i))$$

$$+ \mathbb{P}(\text{mult}(m_i, \mathbf{p}_i) = (0, 0, m_i)|\mathbf{X}_i).$$

Thus, if $\pi > 0$, we have $\mathbb{P}(Z_i = (0, 0, m_i)|\mathbf{X}_i) > \mathbb{P}(\text{mult}(m_i, \mathbf{p}_i) = (0, 0, m_i)|\mathbf{X}_i)$, and the model from equation [4.12] assigns a larger probability to the observation $(0, 0, m_i)$ than the distribution $\text{mult}(m_i, \mathbf{p}_i)$, as expected.

REMARK.– If π is equal to 0, the model from equation [4.12] reduces to the multinomial distribution (in this case, with three categories). □

REMARK.– The identifiability of the ZIM model and the asymptotic properties of the maximum likelihood estimators in this model are established below by assuming that π is constant. However, the proofs are easy to extend to the case where π depends on i (e.g. specified by a logistic model, as we did for the application in section 4.5.5). □

As with the ZIB model, the probabilities p_{1i}, p_{2i} and p_{3i} can be specified by a logistic regression (which, in this case, is multinomial):

$$p_{1i} = \frac{e^{\beta_1^\top \mathbf{X}_i}}{1 + e^{\beta_1^\top \mathbf{X}_i} + e^{\beta_2^\top \mathbf{X}_i}}, \quad p_{2i} = \frac{e^{\beta_2^\top \mathbf{X}_i}}{1 + e^{\beta_1^\top \mathbf{X}_i} + e^{\beta_2^\top \mathbf{X}_i}},$$

$$p_{3i} = 1 - p_{1i} - p_{2i} = \frac{1}{1 + e^{\beta_1^\top \mathbf{X}_i} + e^{\beta_2^\top \mathbf{X}_i}}. \qquad [4.13]$$

The terms β_1 and β_2 are two p-dimensional vectors of unknown parameters. The covariables $\mathbf{X}_i = (1, X_{i2}, \ldots, X_{ip})^\top$ can be either qualitative or quantitative. Let $\beta = (\beta_1^\top, \beta_2^\top)^\top$, and let:

$$\psi = (\pi, \beta_1^\top, \beta_2^\top)^\top$$

be the k-dimensional vector ($k = 1 + 2p$) of all model parameters. For all $i = 1, \ldots, n$, let $J_i = 1_{\{Z_i \neq (0,0,m_i)\}}$ and $h_i(\beta) = 1 + e^{\beta_1^\top \mathbf{X}_i} + e^{\beta_2^\top \mathbf{X}_i}$. We can now easily compute the likelihood of ψ based on the sample of independent observations $(Z_1, \mathbf{X}_1), \ldots, (Z_n, \mathbf{X}_n)$:

$$L_n(\psi) = \prod_{i=1}^{n} \left(\pi + (1 - \pi) p_{1i}^0 p_{2i}^0 p_{3i}^{m_i} \right)^{1 - J_i}$$

$$\times \left((1 - \pi) \frac{m_i!}{Z_{1i}! Z_{2i}! Z_{3i}!} p_{1i}^{Z_{1i}} p_{2i}^{Z_{2i}} p_{3i}^{Z_{3i}} \right)^{J_i}$$

$$= \prod_{i=1}^{n} \left(\pi + (1 - \pi) \frac{1}{(h_i(\beta))^{m_i}} \right)^{1 - J_i}$$

$$\times \left((1 - \pi) \frac{m_i!}{Z_{1i}! Z_{2i}! Z_{3i}!} \frac{e^{Z_{1i} \beta_1^\top \mathbf{X}_i} e^{Z_{2i} \beta_2^\top \mathbf{X}_i}}{(h_i(\beta))^{m_i}} \right)^{J_i}.$$

This gives us the log-likelihood of ψ:

$$\ell_n(\psi) := \sum_{i=1}^{n} \ell_{[i]}(\psi)$$

$$= \sum_{i=1}^{n} \left\{ (1 - J_i) \ln \left(\pi + (1 - \pi) \frac{1}{(h_i(\beta))^{m_i}} \right) \right.$$

$$+ J_i \left[\ln \left(\frac{m_i!}{Z_{1i}! Z_{2i}! Z_{3i}!} \right) - m_i \ln h_i(\beta) \right.$$

$$\left. \left. + Z_{1i} \beta_1^\top \mathbf{X}_i + Z_{2i} \beta_2^\top \mathbf{X}_i + \ln(1 - \pi) \right] \right\}.$$

The maximum likelihood estimator $\hat{\psi}_n := (\hat{\pi}, \hat{\beta}_1^\top, \hat{\beta}_2^\top)^\top$ of ψ is obtained by solving the equation:

$$\frac{\partial}{\partial \psi} \ell_n(\psi) \Big|_{\psi = \hat{\psi}_n} = 0. \tag{4.14}$$

In [DIA 18], the Newton–Raphson algorithm is used to find an approximate solution of equation [4.14]. Below, we shall write $\dot{\ell}_n(\psi) = \frac{\partial}{\partial \psi} \ell_n(\psi)$.

4.5.3. Identifiability

The ZIM model is identifiable. To show this, we need to introduce some notation and regularity conditions. These conditions will be used in the proofs of the identifiability and the asymptotic properties of the maximum likelihood estimator $\hat{\psi}_n$.

REMARK.– The notation introduced below is only used to help follow the proof of the asymptotic results (section 4.5.4). Readers can safely ignore this notation without detracting from the rest of the book. □

4.5.3.1. Notation

In the following, $\mathbf{1}_n$ denotes the n-dimensional row vector for which every component is equal to 1. We will also write $0_{(a,b)}$ for the $(a \times b)$ matrix of zeros. We recall that $k = 1 + 2p$. We define the following matrices:

$$\mathbb{X} = \begin{pmatrix} 1 & 1 & \cdots & 1 \\ X_{12} & X_{22} & \cdots & X_{n2} \\ \vdots & \vdots & \ddots & \vdots \\ X_{1p} & X_{2p} & \cdots & X_{np} \end{pmatrix} \quad \text{and} \quad \mathbb{V} = \begin{pmatrix} \mathbf{1}_n & 0_{(1,n)} & 0_{(1,n)} \\ 0_{(p,n)} & \mathbb{X} & 0_{(p,n)} \\ 0_{(p,n)} & 0_{(p,n)} & \mathbb{X} \end{pmatrix},$$

which have sizes $(p \times n)$ and $(k \times 3n)$, respectively.

For all $i = 1, \ldots, n$, let $k_i(\psi) = \pi \left[(h_i(\beta))^{m_i+1} - h_i(\beta) \right] + h_i(\beta)$ (we recall the notation $h_i(\beta) = 1 + e^{\beta_1^\top \mathbf{X}_i} + e^{\beta_2^\top \mathbf{X}_i}$). We now define:

$$A_i(\psi) = \frac{(h_i(\beta))^{m_i} - 1}{\pi \left[(h_i(\beta))^{m_i} - 1 \right] + 1} (1 - J_i) - \frac{1}{1 - \pi} J_i,$$

$$B_{i,\ell}(\psi) = -(1 - \pi) \frac{m_i e^{\beta_\ell^\top \mathbf{X}_i}}{k_i(\psi)} (1 - J_i)$$

$$+ \left(-\frac{m_i e^{\beta_\ell^\top \mathbf{X}_i}}{h_i(\beta)} + Z_{\ell i} \right) J_i, \quad \ell = 1, 2,$$

and write $C(\psi) = (C_j(\psi))_{1 \le j \le 3n}$ for the $3n$-dimensional column vector given by:

$$C(\psi) = (A_1(\psi), \ldots, A_n(\psi), B_{1,1}(\psi), \ldots, B_{n,1}(\psi), B_{1,2}(\psi), \ldots, B_{n,2}(\psi))^\top.$$

After a few calculations, it can be shown that the score equation from equation [4.14] may be rewritten in the form:

$$\dot{\ell}_n(\psi) = \mathbb{V}C(\psi) = 0.$$

Given an $(a \times b)$ matrix $A = (A_{ij})_{1 \le i \le a, 1 \le j \le b}$, let $A_{\bullet j}$ be the j-th column $(j = 1, \ldots, b)$, i.e. $A_{\bullet j} = (A_{1j}, \ldots, A_{aj})^\top$. Then, the score from equation [4.14] can be rewritten as follows, which will be useful for our proofs:

$$\dot{\ell}_n(\psi) = \sum_{j=1}^{3n} \mathbb{V}_{\bullet j} C_j(\psi).$$

Finally, let $\mathbb{D}(\psi) = (\mathbb{D}_{ij}(\psi))_{1 \le i, j \le 3n}$ be the $(3n \times 3n)$ matrix defined by the following blocks:

$$\mathbb{D}(\psi) = \begin{pmatrix} \mathbb{D}_1(\psi) & \mathbb{D}_4(\psi) & \mathbb{D}_5(\psi) \\ \mathbb{D}_4(\psi) & \mathbb{D}_2(\psi) & \mathbb{D}_6(\psi) \\ \mathbb{D}_5(\psi) & \mathbb{D}_6(\psi) & \mathbb{D}_3(\psi) \end{pmatrix},$$

where $\mathbb{D}_1(\psi), \ldots, \mathbb{D}_6(\psi)$ are the $(n \times n)$ diagonal matrices with i-th diagonal term:

$$\mathbb{D}_{1,ii}(\psi) = \left(\frac{(h_i(\beta))^{m_i} - 1}{\pi \left[(h_i(\beta))^{m_i} - 1 \right] + 1} \right)^2 (1 - J_i) + \frac{1}{(1 - \pi)^2} J_i,$$

$$\mathbb{D}_{\ell+1,ii}(\psi)$$
$$= \frac{(1 - \pi)(1 - J_i)e^{\beta_\ell^\top \mathbf{X}_i} \left((k_i(\psi) - e^{\beta_\ell^\top \mathbf{X}_i}(\pi[(m_i + 1)(h_i(\beta))^{m_i} - 1] + 1) \right)}{(k_i(\psi))^2}$$
$$- \frac{m_i J_i e^{\beta_\ell^\top \mathbf{X}_i} \left(h_i(\beta) - e^{\beta_\ell^\top \mathbf{X}_i} \right)}{(h_i(\beta))^2}, \quad \ell = 1, 2,$$

$$\mathbb{D}_{\ell+3,ii}(\psi) = - \frac{(1 - J_i)m_i e^{\beta_\ell^\top \mathbf{X}_i}(h_i(\beta))^{m_i+1}}{(k_i(\psi))^2}, \quad \ell = 1, 2,$$

$$\mathbb{D}_{6,ii}(\psi) = - \frac{(1 - \pi)(1 - J_i)m_i e^{\beta_1^\top \mathbf{X}_i} e^{\beta_2^\top \mathbf{X}_i} \left(\pi[(h_i(\beta))^{m_i} - 1] + 1 \right)}{(k_i(\psi))^2}$$
$$- \frac{J_i m_i e^{\beta_1^\top \mathbf{X}_i} e^{\beta_2^\top \mathbf{X}_i}}{(h_i(\psi))^2}.$$

Let

$$\ddot{\ell}_n(\psi) = \frac{\partial^2}{\partial \psi \partial \psi^\top} \ell_n(\psi)$$

be the $(k \times k)$ matrix of second derivatives of $\ell_n(\psi)$. After some rather tedious calculations, we find:

$$\ddot{\ell}_n(\psi) = -\mathbb{V}\mathbb{D}(\psi)\mathbb{V}^\top.$$

REMARK.– The vector $C(\psi)$ and the matrices $\mathbb{X}$, $\mathbb{V}$ and $\mathbb{D}(\psi)$ depend on n. However, this dependence is omitted to lighten the notation. □

4.5.3.2. Regularity conditions

The regularity conditions stated by [DIA 18] are as follows:

C1 The explanatory variables X_{ij} are bounded and satisfy $\text{var}(X_{ij}) > 0$ for all $i = 1, 2, \ldots$ and $j = 2, \ldots, p$. The X_{ij} $(j = 1, \ldots, p)$ are linearly independent for all $i = 1, 2, \ldots$

$C2$ The space $\mathbf{K}$ of the parameters $\psi = (\pi, \beta_1^\top, \beta_2^\top)^\top$ is a bounded open subset of $]0, 1[\times\mathbb{R}^p \times \mathbb{R}^p$ (in the following, we shall write $\psi_0 := (\pi_0, \beta_{1,0}^\top, \beta_{2,0}^\top)^\top \in \mathbf{K}$ for the true unknown value of the parameter; we do the same for $\beta_0 = (\beta_{1,0}^\top, \beta_{2,0}^\top)^\top$).

$C3$ The matrix

$$\ddot{\ell}_n(\psi) = \frac{\partial^2}{\partial\psi\partial\psi^\top}\ell_n(\psi)$$

of second derivatives of $\ell_n(\psi)$ is negative definite and full-rank for all $n = 1, 2, \ldots$, and $\frac{1}{n}\ddot{\ell}_n(\psi)$ converges to a negative-definite matrix. Let λ_n and Λ_n be the smallest and largest eigenvalues of the matrix $\mathbb{V}\mathbb{D}(\psi_0)\mathbb{V}^\top$, respectively. There exists a strictly positive constant $c_1 < \infty$ such that $\Lambda_n/\lambda_n < c_1$ for all $n = 1, 2, \ldots$. The matrix $\mathbb{V}\mathbb{V}^\top$ is positive definite for all $n = 1, 2, \ldots$, and its smallest eigenvalue $\tilde{\lambda}_n$ tends to $+\infty$ as n tends to $+\infty$.

The following condition is required for the identifiability of the model:

$C4$ For all $i = 1, \ldots, n$, the inequality $m_i \geq 2$ holds.

REMARK.– When applying the ZIM model to the NMES1988 data (see [DIA 18] and section 4.5.1 of this book), the authors consider patients for whom the total number of office visits of types ofnp, opnp or ofp is greater than or equal to 2. The C4 condition is the reason for this choice.   □

REMARK.– In the following, we will assume that every random variable is defined on the same probability space $(\Omega, \mathcal{C}, \mathbb{P})$. Any results established almost surely implicitly refer to this space.   □

The following theorem establishes the identifiability of the ZIM model.

THEOREM.–   If the conditions C1–C4 hold, then the ZIM model from equations [4.12]–[4.13] is identifiable, i.e. if $\ell_{[i]}(\psi) = \ell_{[i]}(\psi^*)$ almost surely, then $\psi = \psi^*$.

REMARK.– The ZIB model, which is a special case of the ZIM model, is identifiable under the same conditions and, in particular, whenever $m_i \geq 2$ for all $i = 1, \ldots, n$. If $m_i = 1$ for all i, then we recall that the ZIB model is not identifiable. This special case is discussed in section 4.3.2.2.   □

4.5.3.3. *Identifiability of the model: proof*

Suppose that $l_{[i]}(\psi) = l_{[i]}(\psi^*)$ almost surely. The conditions C1 and C2 guarantee that there exists $\epsilon > 0$ such that, for all $\mathbf{X}_i$ and all $\psi \in K$, $\epsilon < \mathbb{P}\left(Z_i \neq (0, 0, m_i) | \mathbf{X}_i\right) = (1 - \pi)\left(1 - (h_i(\beta))^{-m_i}\right)$. We can therefore find some element ω^* of Ω satisfying: i) ω^* is not in the negligible set of ω for which $l_{[i]}(\psi) \neq l_{[i]}(\psi^*)$ and ii) $Z_i(\omega^*) \neq (0, 0, m_i)$. Given any such element ω^*, we have that $J_i(\omega^*) = 1$, and the equality $l_{[i]}(\psi) = l_{[i]}(\psi^*)$ becomes:

$$Z_{1i}(\beta_1 - \beta_1^*)^\top \mathbf{X}_i + Z_{2i}(\beta_2 - \beta_2^*)^\top \mathbf{X}_i$$
$$= \ln\left[\left(\frac{h_i(\beta)}{h_i(\beta^*)}\right)^{m_i} \times \left(\frac{1 - \pi^*}{1 - \pi}\right)\right]. \qquad [4.15]$$

The right-hand side of equation [4.15] does not depend on $Z_i = (Z_{1i}, Z_{2i}, Z_{3i})$, so the left-hand side must be constant for any two given values of Z_i. Let us choose, for example, $Z_i = (z_{1i}, z_{2i}, m_i - z_{1i} - z_{2i})$ and $Z_i = (z_{1i}, z_{2i} - 1, m_i - z_{1i} - z_{2i} + 1)$, with $z_{1i}, z_{2i} \geq 1$ (which we can do by condition C4). Equating the left-hand side of equation [4.15] for these two values yields $(\beta_2 - \beta_2^*)^\top \mathbf{X}_i = 0$, and the condition C1 implies that $\beta_2 = \beta_2^*$. A similar argument shows that $\beta_1 = \beta_1^*$. Returning to equation [4.15], we now obtain $\pi = \pi^*$. This shows that $\psi = \psi^*$. □

REMARK.– The proof of the identifiability of the ZIB model when m_i is equal to 1 for all $i = 1, \ldots, n$ whenever the condition $\mathcal{C}$ holds is based on the same ideas as the proof stated above (see [DIO 11]). □

We shall now describe the asymptotic properties of the maximum likelihood estimator $\hat{\psi}_n = (\hat{\pi}, \hat{\beta}_1^\top, \hat{\beta}_2^\top)^\top$ in the ZIM model. These properties were established by [DIA 18].

4.5.4. *Asymptotics*

The maximum likelihood estimator $\hat{\psi}_n := (\hat{\pi}, \hat{\beta}_1^\top, \hat{\beta}_2^\top)^\top$ is strongly consistent and asymptotically normally distributed. These results are part of the following theorem. Below, I_k denotes the identity matrix of order k. We also write $\widehat{\Sigma}_n = \mathbb{V}\mathbb{D}(\hat{\psi}_n)\mathbb{V}^\top$.

THEOREM.– As n tends to infinity, $\hat{\psi}_n$ converges a.s. to ψ_0 and $\widehat{\Sigma}_n^{\frac{1}{2}}(\hat{\psi}_n - \psi_0)$ converges in distribution to the Gaussian vector $\mathcal{N}(0, I_k)$.

4.5.4.1. *Strong consistency: proof*

Let us begin by stating a lemma that will help us to prove the theorem. The proof of this lemma is given in the appendix of this section.

LEMMA.– Let $\phi_n : \mathbb{R}^k \longrightarrow \mathbb{R}^k$ be the function defined by $\phi_n(\psi) = \psi + (\mathbb{V}D(\psi_0)\mathbb{V}^\top)^{-1}\dot{\ell}_n(\psi)$. There exists an open ball $B(\psi_0, r) = \{\psi \in \mathbb{R}^k; \|\psi - \psi_0\| < r\}$ (where $r > 0$) and a constant $c \in\ ]0, 1[$ such that:

$$\|\phi_n(\psi) - \phi_n(\tilde{\psi})\| \leq c\|\psi - \tilde{\psi}\| \text{ for all } \psi, \tilde{\psi} \in B(\psi_0, r). \qquad [4.16]$$

This lemma will allow us to show that the maximum likelihood estimator is strongly consistent. First, we recall the following definition.

Let X be a random variable and $(X_n)_{n \in \mathbb{N}}$ be a sequence of random variables in $\mathbb{R}^k$ defined on the same probability space $(\Omega, \mathcal{C}, \mathbb{P})$. We say that the sequence $(X_n)_{n \in \mathbb{N}}$ converges a.s. to X if $\lim_{n \to \infty} X_n(\omega) = X(\omega)$ for all $\omega \in \Omega \backslash \mathcal{N}$, where $\mathcal{N}$ is a negligible subset of Ω (i.e. which satisfies $\mathbb{P}(\mathcal{N}) = 0$).

Let η_n be the function defined by $\eta_n(\psi) = \psi - \phi_n(\psi) = -(\mathbb{V}D(\psi_0)\mathbb{V}^\top)^{-1}\dot{\ell}_n(\psi)$. Then, $\eta_n(\psi_0)$ converges a.s. to 0 as n tends to infinity. To see this, we observe that:

$$\eta_n(\psi_0) = \left(\frac{1}{n}\ddot{\ell}_n(\psi_0)\right)^{-1} \cdot \left(\frac{1}{n}\dot{\ell}_n(\psi_0)\right).$$

By condition C3, $\left(\frac{1}{n}\ddot{\ell}_n(\psi_0)\right)^{-1}$ converges to some matrix Σ. Furthermore:

$$\frac{1}{n}\dot{\ell}_n(\psi_0) = \frac{1}{n}\mathbb{V}C(\psi_0) = \begin{pmatrix} \frac{1}{n}\sum_{i=1}^n A_i(\psi_0) \\ \frac{1}{n}\sum_{i=1}^n X_{i1}B_{i,1}(\psi_0) \\ \vdots \\ \frac{1}{n}\sum_{i=1}^n X_{ip}B_{i,1}(\psi_0) \\ \frac{1}{n}\sum_{i=1}^n X_{i1}B_{i,2}(\psi_0) \\ \vdots \\ \frac{1}{n}\sum_{i=1}^n X_{ip}B_{i,2}(\psi_0) \end{pmatrix}$$

converges a.s. to 0 as n tends to infinity. Indeed, for all $i = 1, \dots, n$, we note that $\mathbb{E}[A_i(\psi_0)] = \mathbb{E}[\mathbb{E}[A_i(\psi_0)|\mathbf{X}_i]]$, where:

$$\mathbb{E}[A_i(\psi_0)|\mathbf{X}_i] = \frac{(h_i(\beta_0))^{m_i} - 1}{\pi_0[(h_i(\beta_0))^{m_i} - 1] + 1} \mathbb{E}\left[1 - J_i|\mathbf{X}_i\right] - \frac{1}{1 - \pi_0}\mathbb{E}\left[J_i|\mathbf{X}_i\right].$$

Now, we have:

$$\mathbb{E}\left[J_i|\mathbf{X}_i\right] = \mathbb{P}(Z_i \neq (0,0,m_i)|\mathbf{X}_i) = (1 - \pi_0)\left(1 - \frac{1}{(h_i(\beta_0))^{m_i}}\right),$$

so:

$$\mathbb{E}[A_i(\psi_0)|\mathbf{X}_i] = \frac{(h_i(\beta_0))^{m_i} - 1}{\pi_0[(h_i(\beta_0))^{m_i} - 1] + 1}\left[\pi_0 + (1 - \pi_0)\frac{1}{(h_i(\beta_0))^{m_i}}\right]$$

$$- \left(1 - \frac{1}{(h_i(\beta_0))^{m_i}}\right)$$

$$= 0.$$

Hence, $\mathbb{E}[A_i(\psi_0)] = 0$. Next, for all $i = 1, \dots, n$:

$$\text{var}(A_i(\psi_0)) = \mathbb{E}[\text{var}(A_i(\psi_0)|\mathbf{X}_i)] + \text{var}(\mathbb{E}[A_i(\psi_0)|\mathbf{X}_i])$$

$$= \mathbb{E}[\text{var}(A_i(\psi_0)|\mathbf{X}_i)]$$

$$\leq c_2 := \mathbb{E}\left[\left(\frac{(h_i(\beta_0))^{m_i}}{(1 - \pi_0)\{\pi_0[(h_i(\beta_0))^{m_i} - 1] + 1\}}\right)^2\right].$$

The conditions C1, C2 and C4 guarantee that $c_2 < \infty$, so:

$$\sum_{i=1}^{\infty} \frac{\text{var}(A_i(\psi_0))}{i^2} \leq c_2 \sum_{i=1}^{\infty} \frac{1}{i^2} < \infty.$$

Kolmogorov's strong law of large numbers (see [JIA 10], Theorem 6.7) then guarantees that:

$$\frac{1}{n}\sum_{i=1}^{n}\{A_i(\psi_0) - \mathbb{E}\left[A_i(\psi_0)\right]\} = \frac{1}{n}\sum_{i=1}^{n} A_i(\psi_0)$$

converges a.s. to 0 as n tends to infinity. Similarly, for all $i = 1, \ldots, n$ and $j = 1, \ldots, p$, we have that $\mathbb{E}[X_{ij}B_{i,1}(\psi_0)] = \mathbb{E}[X_{ij}\mathbb{E}[B_{i,1}(\psi_0)|\mathbf{X}_i]]$, where:

$$\mathbb{E}[B_{i,1}(\psi_0)|\mathbf{X}_i] = -(1 - \pi_0)\frac{m_i e^{\beta_{1,0}^\top \mathbf{X}_i}}{k_i(\psi_0)}\mathbb{E}\left[1 - J_i|\mathbf{X}_i\right]$$

$$- \frac{m_i e^{\beta_{1,0}^\top \mathbf{X}_i}}{h_i(\beta_0)}\mathbb{E}\left[J_i|\mathbf{X}_i\right] + \mathbb{E}\left[J_i Z_{1i}|\mathbf{X}_i\right]$$

and

$$\mathbb{E}\left[J_i Z_{1i}|\mathbf{X}_i\right] = (1 - \pi_0)m_i \frac{e^{\beta_{1,0}^\top \mathbf{X}_i}}{h_i(\beta_0)}.$$

It is easy to check that $\mathbb{E}[B_{i,1}(\psi_0)|\mathbf{X}_i] = 0$, and so $\mathbb{E}[X_{ij}B_{i,1}(\psi_0)] = 0$. Using a similar reasoning to the above, we can also show that:

$$\sum_{i=1}^{\infty} \frac{\text{var}(X_{ij}B_{i,1}(\psi_0))}{i^2} < \infty.$$

Hence, $\frac{1}{n}\sum_{i=1}^{n} X_{ij}B_{i,1}(\psi_0)$ converges a.s. to 0 as n tends to infinity. A similar result can be shown for $\frac{1}{n}\sum_{i=1}^{n} X_{ij}B_{i,2}(\psi_0)$ by reasoning analogously. Finally, $\frac{1}{n}\dot{\ell}_n(\psi_0)$ and $\eta_n(\psi_0)$ converge a.s. to 0 as n tends to infinity.

Now, let ϵ be a strictly positive number. The fact that $\eta_n(\psi_0)$ converges almost surely implies that, for almost every $\omega \in \Omega$, there exists an integer $n(\epsilon, \omega)$ such that, if $n \geq n(\epsilon, \omega)$, then $\|\eta_n(\psi_0)\| \leq \epsilon$, or equivalently $0 \in B(\eta_n(\psi_0), \epsilon)$. In particular, let $\epsilon = (1 - c)s$, where $c \in]0, 1[$ is as in the preparatory lemma stated above. The function ϕ_n satisfies the Lipschitz condition in equation [4.16], so Lemma 2 from [GOU 81] guarantees that there exists an element of $B(\psi_0, s)$ (denoted $\widehat{\psi}_n$) such that $\eta_n(\widehat{\psi}_n) = 0$, i.e. $(\mathbb{V}\mathbf{D}(\psi_0)\mathbf{V}^\top)^{-1}\dot{\ell}_n(\widehat{\psi}_n) = 0$. Condition C3 implies that $\dot{\ell}_n(\widehat{\psi}_n) = 0$ and that $\widehat{\psi}_n$ is the unique value that maximizes ℓ_n.

In summary, we have shown that, for almost every $\omega \in \Omega$ and for all $s > 0$, there exists an integer $n(s, \omega)$ such that, if $n \geq n(s, \omega)$, then the maximum likelihood estimator $\widehat{\psi}_n$ exists and $\|\widehat{\psi}_n - \psi_0\| \leq s$ (i.e. $\widehat{\psi}_n$ converges a.s. to ψ_0). $\qquad\square$

4.5.4.2. *Asymptotic normality: proof*

By considering the Taylor expansion of the score function, we have:

$$0 = \dot{\ell}_n(\widehat{\psi}_n) = \dot{\ell}_n(\psi_0) + \ddot{\ell}_n(\widetilde{\psi}_n)(\widehat{\psi}_n - \psi_0),$$

where $\widetilde{\psi}_n$ belongs to the segment $[\widehat{\psi}_n, \psi_0]$. Hence, $\dot{\ell}_n(\psi_0) = -\ddot{\ell}_n(\widetilde{\psi}_n)(\widehat{\psi}_n - \psi_0)$. Let $\widetilde{\Sigma}_n := -\ddot{\ell}_n(\widetilde{\psi}_n) = \mathbb{V}\mathbb{D}(\widetilde{\psi}_n)\mathbb{V}^\top$ and $\Sigma_{n,0} := \mathbb{V}\mathbb{D}(\psi_0)\mathbb{V}^\top$. Then:

$$\widehat{\Sigma}_n^{\frac{1}{2}}(\widehat{\psi}_n - \psi_0) = \left[\widehat{\Sigma}_n^{\frac{1}{2}}\widetilde{\Sigma}_n^{-\frac{1}{2}}\right]\left[\widetilde{\Sigma}_n^{-\frac{1}{2}}\Sigma_{n,0}^{\frac{1}{2}}\right]\Sigma_{n,0}^{-\frac{1}{2}}\left(\widetilde{\Sigma}_n(\widehat{\psi}_n - \psi_0)\right). \quad [4.17]$$

The terms $[\widehat{\Sigma}_n^{\frac{1}{2}}\widetilde{\Sigma}_n^{-\frac{1}{2}}]$ and $[\widetilde{\Sigma}_n^{-\frac{1}{2}}\Sigma_{n,0}^{\frac{1}{2}}]$ in equation [4.17] converge a.s. to I_k. For instance, let us show that $\|\widetilde{\Sigma}_n^{-\frac{1}{2}}\Sigma_{n,0}^{\frac{1}{2}} - I_k\| \xrightarrow{a.s.} 0$ as n tends to infinity. First, we observe that:

$$\left\|\widetilde{\Sigma}_n^{-\frac{1}{2}}\Sigma_{n,0}^{\frac{1}{2}} - I_k\right\| = \left\|\widetilde{\Sigma}_n^{-\frac{1}{2}}[\Sigma_{n,0}^{\frac{1}{2}} - \widetilde{\Sigma}_n^{\frac{1}{2}}]\right\|$$

$$\leq \left\|\widetilde{\Sigma}_n^{-\frac{1}{2}}\right\|\left\|\Sigma_{n,0}^{\frac{1}{2}} - \widetilde{\Sigma}_n^{\frac{1}{2}}\right\|$$

$$\leq \Lambda_n^{\frac{1}{2}}\left\|\widetilde{\Sigma}_n^{-\frac{1}{2}}\right\|\left\|\Lambda_n^{-\frac{1}{2}}\left(\Sigma_{n,0}^{\frac{1}{2}} - \widetilde{\Sigma}_n^{\frac{1}{2}}\right)\right\|$$

and

$$\Lambda_n^{-1}\left\|\Sigma_{n,0} - \widetilde{\Sigma}_n\right\| = \Lambda_n^{-1}\left\|\mathbb{V}(\mathbb{D}(\psi_0) - \mathbb{D}(\widetilde{\psi}_n))\mathbb{V}^\top\right\|.$$

We know that $\widetilde{\psi}_n$ converges a.s. to ψ_0. Therefore, let ω be an element of Ω for which this convergence holds. By the same arguments as in the proof of the introductory lemma, we can show that, for all $\epsilon > 0$, there exists $n(\epsilon, \omega) \in \mathbb{N}$ such that, if $n \geq n(\epsilon, \omega)$, then $\Lambda_n^{-1}\|\mathbb{V}(\mathbb{D}(\psi_0) - \mathbb{D}(\widetilde{\psi}_n))\mathbb{V}^\top\| \leq \epsilon$. Hence, $\Lambda_n^{-1}\|\mathbb{V}(\mathbb{D}(\psi_0) - \mathbb{D}(\widetilde{\psi}_n))\mathbb{V}^\top\|$ converges a.s. to 0. By the continuity of the function $A \mapsto A^{\frac{1}{2}}$, $\|\Lambda_n^{-\frac{1}{2}}(\Sigma_{n,0}^{\frac{1}{2}} - \widetilde{\Sigma}_n^{\frac{1}{2}})\|$ also converges a.s. to 0.

Furthermore, for sufficiently large n, there exists $c_3 \in (0, \infty)$ such that $\Lambda_n^{\frac{1}{2}}\|\widetilde{\Sigma}_n^{-\frac{1}{2}}\| \leq c_3\Lambda_n^{\frac{1}{2}}/\lambda_n^{\frac{1}{2}} < c_3 c_1^{\frac{1}{2}}$ holds almost surely (by condition C3).

We conclude that $\|\widetilde{\Sigma}_n^{-\frac{1}{2}}\Sigma_{n,0}^{\frac{1}{2}} - I_k\|$ converges a.s. to 0. The fact that $\|\widehat{\Sigma}_n^{\frac{1}{2}}\widetilde{\Sigma}_n^{-\frac{1}{2}} - I_k\|$ converges a.s. to 0 can be shown analogously.

It now simply remains to be shown that $\Sigma_{n,0}^{-\frac{1}{2}}(\widetilde{\Sigma}_n(\widehat{\psi}_n - \psi_0))$ converges in distribution to the Gaussian vector $\mathcal{N}(0, I_k)$. We observe that:

$$\Sigma_{n,0}^{-\frac{1}{2}}(\widetilde{\Sigma}_n(\widehat{\psi}_n - \psi_0)) = \Sigma_{n,0}^{-\frac{1}{2}} \sum_{j=1}^{3n} \mathbf{V}_{\bullet j} C_j(\psi_0).$$

We can apply the central limit theorem stated in [EIC 66] to deduce that this convergence holds if the following three conditions are satisfied:

1) $\max_{1 \leq j \leq 3n} \mathbf{V}_{\bullet j}^{\top}(\mathbf{V}\mathbf{V}^{\top})^{-1}\mathbf{V}_{\bullet j} \to 0$ as n tends to infinity,

2) $\sup_{1 \leq j \leq 3n} \mathbb{E}[C_j(\psi_0)^2 1_{\{|C_j(\psi_0)|>c\}}] \to 0$ as c tends to infinity,

3) $\inf_{1 \leq j \leq 3n} \mathbb{E}[C_j(\psi_0)^2] > 0$.

We can verify that condition 1) is satisfied by observing that:

$$0 < \max_{1 \leq j \leq 3n} \mathbf{V}_{\bullet j}^{\top}(\mathbf{V}\mathbf{V}^{\top})^{-1}\mathbf{V}_{\bullet j}$$

$$\leq \max_{1 \leq j \leq 3n} \|\mathbf{V}_{\bullet j}\|^2\|(\mathbf{V}\mathbf{V}^{\top})^{-1}\| = \max_{1 \leq j \leq 3n} \frac{\|\mathbf{V}_{\bullet j}\|^2}{\widetilde{\lambda}_n},$$

and that $\|\mathbf{V}_{\bullet j}\|$ is bounded, by C1. Furthermore, $1/\widetilde{\lambda}_n$ tends to 0 as n tends to infinity, by C3. To show condition 2), we note that the quantities $C_j(\psi_0)$, $j = 1, \ldots, 3n$ are bounded by C1, C2 and C4. Finally, we note that $\mathbb{E}[C_j(\psi_0)^2] = \text{var}(C_j(\psi_0))$, since $\mathbb{E}[C_j(\psi_0)] = 0$, $j = 1, \ldots, 3n$. For $j \in \{1, \ldots, n\}$, $C_j(\psi_0) = A_j(\psi_0)$. Thus, $\text{var}(C_j(\psi_0)) = \text{var}(A_j(\psi_0)) = \mathbb{E}[\text{var}(A_j(\psi_0)|\mathbf{X}_j)]$. Then:

$$\text{var}(A_j(\psi_0)|\mathbf{X}_j) = \left(\frac{(h_j(\beta_0))^{m_j}}{(1 - \pi_0)[\pi_0((h_j(\beta_0))^{m_j} - 1) + 1]}\right)^2 \text{var}(J_j|\mathbf{X}_j)$$

$$= \left(\frac{(h_j(\beta_0))^{m_j}}{(1 - \pi_0)[\pi_0((h_j(\beta_0))^{m_j} - 1) + 1]}\right)^2$$

$$\times \mathbb{P}(Z_j \neq (0, 0, m_j)|\mathbf{X}_j) \cdot (1 - \mathbb{P}(Z_j \neq (0, 0, m_j)|\mathbf{X}_j))$$

$$= \left(\frac{(h_j(\beta_0))^{m_j}}{(1 - \pi_0)[\pi_0((h_j(\beta_0))^{m_j} - 1) + 1]} \right)^2$$

$$\times \left((1 - \pi_0)(1 - \frac{1}{(h_j(\beta_0))^{m_j}}) \right)$$

$$\times \left(\pi_0 + (1 - \pi_0)\frac{1}{(h_j(\beta_0))^{m_j}} \right),$$

and so $\mathrm{var}(A_j(\psi_0)|\mathbf{X}_j) > 0$ for all $j = 1, \ldots, n$, by C1, C2 and C4. Thus, $\mathrm{var}(C_j(\psi_0)) > 0$ for all $j = 1, \ldots, n$. We can show that $\mathrm{var}(C_j(\psi_0)) > 0$ for all $j = 1, \ldots, 3n$ analogously, and so condition 3) also holds.

In summary, we have shown that $\Sigma_{n,0}^{-\frac{1}{2}}(\widetilde{\Sigma}_n(\widehat{\psi}_n - \psi_0))$ converges in distribution to $\mathcal{N}(0, I_k)$. By applying this result together with Slutsky's theorem to equation [4.17], we deduce that $\widehat{\Sigma}_n^{\frac{1}{2}}(\widehat{\psi}_n - \psi_0)$ converges in distribution to the Gaussian vector $\mathcal{N}(0, I_k)$. $\qquad\square$

4.5.4.3. Technical appendix

We shall now give a proof of the preparatory lemma stated at the beginning of section 4.5.4. The property from equation [4.16] necessarily holds if we can show that $\left\| \frac{\partial \phi_n(\psi)}{\partial \psi^\top} \right\| \leq c$ for all $\psi \in B(\psi_0, r)$. First, we observe that:

$$\left\| \frac{\partial \phi_n(\psi)}{\partial \psi^\top} \right\| = \left\| I_k + (\mathrm{V}\mathbb{D}(\psi_0)\mathrm{V}^\top)^{-1}\ddot{l}_n(\psi) \right\|$$

$$= \left\| (\mathrm{V}\mathbb{D}(\psi_0)\mathrm{V}^\top)^{-1}\mathrm{V}(\mathbb{D}(\psi_0) - \mathbb{D}(\psi))\mathrm{V}^\top \right\|$$

$$\leq \left\| (\mathrm{V}\mathbb{D}(\psi_0)\mathrm{V}^\top)^{-1} \right\| \left\| \mathrm{V}(\mathbb{D}(\psi_0) - \mathbb{D}(\psi))\mathrm{V}^\top \right\|$$

$$= \lambda_n^{-1} \left\| \mathrm{V}(\mathbb{D}(\psi_0) - \mathbb{D}(\psi))\mathrm{V}^\top \right\|.$$

We write $\mathcal{I}$ for the set of $(i, j) \in \{1, 2, \ldots, 3n\}^2$ such that $\mathbb{D}_{ij}(\psi_0) \neq 0$. Then:

$$\left\| \mathrm{V}(\mathbb{D}(\psi_0) - \mathbb{D}(\psi))\mathrm{V}^\top \right\| = \left\| \sum_{i=1}^{3n}\sum_{j=1}^{3n} \mathrm{V}_{\bullet i}\mathrm{V}_{\bullet j}^\top(\mathbb{D}_{ij}(\psi) - \mathbb{D}_{ij}(\psi_0)) \right\|$$

$$\leq \sum_{(i,j)\in\mathcal{I}} \left\| \mathrm{V}_{\bullet i}\mathrm{V}_{\bullet j}^\top\mathbb{D}_{ij}(\psi_0) \right\| \left| \frac{\mathbb{D}_{ij}(\psi) - \mathbb{D}_{ij}(\psi_0)}{\mathbb{D}_{ij}(\psi_0)} \right|.$$

Given conditions C1 and C2, there exists a strictly positive constant c_4 such that $|\mathbb{D}_{ij}(\psi_0)| > c_4$ for all $(i,j) \in \mathcal{I}$. For example, we consider the case where $\mathbb{D}_{ij}(\psi_0)$ coincides with one of the $\mathbb{D}_{4,\ell\ell}(\psi_0)$, for $\ell \in \{1, \ldots, n\}$. Then:

$$|\mathbb{D}_{4,\ell\ell}(\psi)| = \frac{m_\ell e^{\beta_1^\top \mathbf{X}_\ell}(h_\ell(\beta))^{m_\ell-1}}{(\pi[(h_\ell(\beta))^{m_\ell} - 1] + 1)^2} > \frac{m_{\mathbf{X}}}{(1 + 2M_{\mathbf{X}})^{2m_\ell}},$$

where $m_{\mathbf{X}} := \min_{\beta,\mathbf{X}} e^{\beta^\top \mathbf{X}}$ and $M_{\mathbf{X}} := \max_{\beta,\mathbf{X}} e^{\beta^\top \mathbf{X}}$. By conditions C1, C2 and C4, there exists a strictly positive constant d_4 such that $\frac{m_{\mathbf{X}}}{(1+2M_{\mathbf{X}})^{2m_\ell}} > d_4$. Similarly, for $i = 1, \ldots, 6$, we can show that $|\mathbb{D}_{i,\ell\ell}(\psi)| > d_i$ for a suitable constant d_i. If we set $c_4 = \min_{1 \le i \le 6} d_i$, then $|\mathbb{D}_{ij}(\psi_0)| > c_4$ for all $(i,j) \in \mathcal{I}$. Furthermore, $\mathbb{D}_{ij}(\cdot)$ is uniformly continuous on $\mathbf{K}$, so, for all $\epsilon > 0$, there exists $r > 0$ such that, for all $\psi \in B(\psi_0, r)$, $|\mathbb{D}_{ij}(\psi) - \mathbb{D}_{ij}(\psi_0)| < \epsilon$. We therefore have that:

$$\left\| \mathbf{V}(\mathbb{D}(\psi_0) - \mathbb{D}(\psi))\mathbf{V}^\top \right\| \le \frac{\epsilon}{c_4} \sum_{(i,j) \in \mathcal{I}} \left\| \mathbf{V}_{\bullet i}\mathbf{V}_{\bullet j}^\top \mathbb{D}_{ij}(\psi_0) \right\|$$

$$= \frac{\epsilon}{c_4}\text{trace}\left(\mathbf{V}\mathbb{D}(\psi_0)\mathbf{V}^\top \right)$$

$$\le \frac{\epsilon}{c_4}k\Lambda_n.$$

This then implies that $\left\| \frac{\partial\phi_n(\psi)}{\partial\psi^\top} \right\| \le \frac{\epsilon k\Lambda_n}{c_4\lambda_n} < \frac{\epsilon k c_1}{c_4}$. Now, setting $\epsilon = c\frac{c_4}{kc_1}$, for $c \in]0, 1[$, we find that $\left\| \frac{\partial\phi_n(\psi)}{\partial\psi^\top} \right\| \le c$ for all $\psi \in B(\psi_0, r)$, which completes the proof. $\square$

4.5.5. Application to healthcare economics

Let us return once again to the NMES1988 data and the problem stated in section 4.5.1. Our objective is to establish a simultaneous model of the consumption of three types of healthcare. For each of the 3,224 patients, we know the number Z_{1i} of office visits to a non-physician (ofnp), the number Z_{2i} of outpatient appointments with a non-physician (opnp) and the number Z_{3i} of office visits to a physician (ofp). The data analysis performed in section 4.5.1 suggests that there is an inflated number of observations of type $Z_i = (0, 0, m_i)$, where $Z_i := (Z_{1i}, Z_{2i}, Z_{3i})$ and m_i represents the total number of times the i-th patient sought healthcare of type ofnp, opnp or ofp over the duration of the study. In [DIA 18], the authors propose to use the following ZIM model for Z_i:

$$Z_i \sim \begin{cases} (0,0,m_i) & \text{with probability } \pi_i \\ \text{mult}(m_i, \mathbf{p}_i) & \text{with probability } 1 - \pi_i \end{cases}$$

where the probabilities $\mathbf{p}_i = (p_{1i}, p_{2i}, p_{3i})$ are specified by a multinomial logistic model:

$$p_{1i} = \frac{e^{\beta_1^\top \mathbf{X}_i}}{1 + e^{\beta_1^\top \mathbf{X}_i} + e^{\beta_2^\top \mathbf{X}_i}}, \quad p_{2i} = \frac{e^{\beta_2^\top \mathbf{X}_i}}{1 + e^{\beta_1^\top \mathbf{X}_i} + e^{\beta_2^\top \mathbf{X}_i}},$$

$$p_{3i} = 1 - p_{1i} - p_{2i} = \frac{1}{1 + e^{\beta_1^\top \mathbf{X}_i} + e^{\beta_2^\top \mathbf{X}_i}}.$$

As noted earlier, p_{1i} represents the probability that the i-th patient chooses to visit a non-physician in an office setting (i.e. seeks healthcare of type ofnp) given the choice between the three types of healthcare ofnp, opnp and ofp and assuming that the patient does not systematically avoid healthcare of type ofnp and opnp. The probabilities p_{2i} and p_{3i} have similar interpretations. The value π_i may be interpreted as the probability that the i-th patient systematically avoids visiting non-physicians, whether in an office or outpatient setting.

In this application, π_i may depend on the covariables. We shall model it by a logistic regression:

$$\pi_i = \frac{e^{\gamma^\top \mathbf{W}_i}}{1 + e^{\gamma^\top \mathbf{W}_i}}.$$

First, we shall estimate a ZIM model in which $\mathbf{X}_i$ and $\mathbf{W}_i$ contain all available covariables (health1, health2, numchron, age, gender, fstatus, school, income and med). The Newton–Raphson algorithm is used to derive an approximate solution of the estimation equation [4.14].

The output shown below lists the estimates of the parameters, the "standard errors", the Wald statistic (which tests the nullity of each parameter) and the corresponding p-values. The coefficients [1,] to [10,] (respectively [11,] to [20,] and [21,] to [30,]) correspond to the components of γ (respectively β_1 and β_2).

```
Maximum Likelihood estimation
Newton-Raphson maximisation, 9 iterations
Return code 2: successive function values within
    tolerance limit
Log-Likelihood: -14140.55
30  free parameters
Estimates:
         Estimate Std. error t value  Pr(> t)
  [1,] -0.589449   0.776250   -0.759 0.447640
  [2,]  0.253401   0.141777    1.787 0.073887 .
  [3,]  0.155717   0.216155    0.720 0.471284
  [4,] -0.050798   0.035572   -1.428 0.153284
  [5,]  0.164659   0.095898    1.717 0.085976 .
  [6,] -0.277737   0.103705   -2.678 0.007403 **
  [7,] -0.008539   0.106784   -0.080 0.936266
  [8,] -0.072678   0.014165   -5.131 2.89e-07 ***
  [9,] -0.009066   0.017536   -0.517 0.605157
 [10,]  0.531909   0.162704    3.269 0.001079 **
 [11,] -1.248610   0.289708   -4.310 1.63e-05 ***
 [12,] -0.396494   0.071739   -5.527 3.26e-08 ***
 [13,]  0.322671   0.084017    3.841 0.000123 ***
 [14,] -0.128286   0.016428   -7.809 5.76e-15 ***
 [15,]  0.022117   0.035517    0.623 0.533483
 [16,]  0.184823   0.047366    3.902 9.54e-05 ***
 [17,]  0.203610   0.047860    4.254 2.10e-05 ***
 [18,]  0.007447   0.006546    1.138 0.255269
 [19,] -0.010011   0.006633   -1.509 0.131252
 [20,] -0.036510   0.090085   -0.405 0.685269
 [21,]  2.165172   0.462911    4.677 2.91e-06 ***
 [22,]  0.131013   0.099197    1.321 0.186592
 [23,] -0.390306   0.177727   -2.196 0.028085 *
 [24,] -0.037507   0.024871   -1.508 0.131539
 [25,] -0.553270   0.059143   -9.355  < 2e-16 ***
 [26,] -0.028941   0.074988   -0.386 0.699539
 [27,] -0.239747   0.074548   -3.216 0.001300 **
 [28,] -0.017682   0.010534   -1.679 0.093223 .
 [29,]  0.010995   0.009524    1.154 0.248312
 [30,] -0.398524   0.150691   -2.645 0.008178 **
---
Signif. codes: 0 '***' 0.001'**' 0.01'*' 0.05'.' 0.1 '' 1
```

Next, we shall perform an automatic selection of variables based on the AIC criterion. The ZIM model retained after the selection of variables is stated in Table 4.4.

parameter	variable	estimate	s.e.	Wald test	Pr(>t)	
$\beta_{1,1}$	constant	-1.248440	0.327153	-3.816	0.000136	***
$\beta_{1,2}$	health1	-0.396752	0.071734	-5.531	3.19e-08	***
$\beta_{1,3}$	health2	0.307117	0.078294	3.923	8.76e-05	***
$\beta_{1,4}$	numchron	-0.128615	0.016425	-7.830	4.87e-15	***
$\beta_{1,5}$	age	0.021925	0.039900	0.550	0.582655	
$\beta_{1,6}$	gender	0.184974	0.046684	3.962	7.43e-05	***
$\beta_{1,7}$	fstatus	0.204095	0.046834	4.358	1.31e-05	***
$\beta_{1,8}$	school	0.007483	0.006577	1.138	0.255254	
$\beta_{1,9}$	income	-0.009338	0.006506	-1.435	0.151202	
$\beta_{1,10}$	med	-0.034313	0.090432	-0.379	0.704366	
$\beta_{2,1}$	constant	2.164690	0.465538	4.650	3.32e-06	***
$\beta_{2,2}$	health1	0.130806	0.097185	1.346	0.178319	
$\beta_{2,3}$	health2	-0.405494	0.166065	-2.442	0.014615	*
$\beta_{2,4}$	numchron	-0.037862	0.024914	-1.520	0.128586	
$\beta_{2,5}$	age	-0.553335	0.058814	-9.408	< 2e-16	***
$\beta_{2,6}$	gender	-0.028528	0.073176	-0.390	0.696649	
$\beta_{2,7}$	fstatus	-0.239131	0.072781	-3.286	0.001018	**
$\beta_{2,8}$	school	-0.017676	0.010526	-1.679	0.093101	.
$\beta_{2,9}$	income	0.011618	0.009440	1.231	0.218424	
$\beta_{2,10}$	med	-0.397013	0.148050	-2.682	0.007327	**
γ_1	constant	-0.605712	0.548682	-1.104	0.269619	
γ_2	health1	0.249759	0.137186	1.821	0.068670	.
γ_3	numchron	-0.053888	0.035305	-1.526	0.126922	
γ_4	age	0.165217	0.069555	2.375	0.017532	*
γ_5	gender	-0.269703	0.091465	-2.949	0.003191	**
γ_6	school	-0.073233	0.012854	-5.697	1.22e-08	***
γ_7	med	0.543147	0.160838	3.377	0.000733	***

Table 4.4. *Estimation of the ZIM model on the NMES data*

Analyzing these results gives some interesting insight. The significant variables in the logistic model for π_i (to the 5% level) are age, gender, school and med. The probability that a patient systematically avoids visiting a non-physician (either in an office or in an outpatient setting) increases with age, decreases with education and increases in Medicaid beneficiaries.

In light of the p-values ($1.22 \cdot 10^{-08}$ for school and 0.000733 for med), it seems that low education and income levels are the principal determining factors of the renunciation of healthcare of types ofnp and opnp. In [DEB 97], the authors hypothesize that the education level of the patient reflects his or her awareness of the range of healthcare services available. Lower education levels may be associated with a lack of awareness of existing healthcare options, preventing patients from taking advantage of them. Another hypothesis is that lower education levels are associated with less medical knowledge, which may make it more difficult for some patients to communicate about their state of health and understand the responses given by the medical community, also contributing to the renunciation of healthcare. Finally, social relations and social distance from healthcare practitioners and institutions may render the act of seeking healthcare intimidating to patients with lower levels of education.

The variables health1 and numchron, which measure the state of health of the patients, are not significant to the 5% level in the logistic model for π_i (although only be a relatively small margin). Thus, the most important individual factors of the renunciation of healthcare of types ofnp and opnp appear to relate to the financial means of the patients, which tends to support the hypothesis that the most vulnerable categories of patients are the mostly likely to avoid seeking healthcare.

We note that the selection procedure of the model did not retain the income variable in the logistic model for π_i (and income was also not significant in the linear predictors of p_{1i} and p_{2i}). This observation seems surprising *a priori* and was one of the findings of the analysis performed in [DEB 97] when considering each measure of healthcare consumption individually. One reasonable explanation is that the effect of income levels on healthcare consumption is fully captured by the med variable (indicating eligibility for Medicaid coverage and therefore indirectly representing the patient's income level). In [DEB 97], the authors also propose that the income level of a patient might only affect the type and quality of healthcare sought by the patient rather than the number of appointments.

In patients who do not systematically avoid visiting non-physicians, the probability of seeking an appointment of type ofnp decreases as their state of health (measured by the health1 and numchron variables) deteriorates. Since the variables health1 and numchron are not significant in the linear predictor of p_{2i} (the probability of visiting a non-physician in an outpatient setting), the decrease in the probability of seeking an appointment of type ofnp in patients with deteriorating health is necessarily accompanied by an increase in the probability p_{3i} of visiting a physician in an office setting. This observation is intuitively reasonable, since patients in deteriorating health can be expected to prioritize more medically oriented appointments.

The probability of visiting a non-physician in an outpatient setting decreases with age. Since the age variable is not significant in the linear predictor of p_{1i}, this decrease is necessarily accompanied by an increase in the probability p_{3i} of visiting a physician in an office setting. This observation was also reported by [DEB 97]. The authors offer the explanation that elderly patients who live further away from urban centers may experience more difficulties in attending outpatient appointments in a hospital or a clinic. These mobility obstacles may therefore lead them to prefer office visits to a physician located in closer proximity to their homes.

Male patients appear to be more likely than female patients to systematically avoid visiting non-physicians (whether in an office or in an outpatient setting). For office visits, male patients also seem to prefer physicians over non-physicians. This observation is consistent with the findings of [DEB 97], who attribute this phenomenon to the tendency of male patients to only seek healthcare as the last option, once medical care becomes unavoidable.

Hence, on the NMES1988 data, the conclusions of the ZIM model are consistent with the findings of other models that only consider a single measure of healthcare consumption. However, by considering multiple measures simultaneously, the ZIM model improves our understanding of the determining factors of healthcare consumption and renunciation by revealing how the act of choosing one type of healthcare changes the behavior of patients toward the other types of healthcare available to them.

References

[ANT 92] ANTONIADIS A., BERRUYER J., CARMONA R., *Régression non linéaire et applications*, Economica, 1992.

[AZA 06] AZAÏS J.-M., BARDET J.-M., *Le Modèle Linéaire par l'exemple Régression, Analyse de la Variance et Plans d'Expériences Illustrations numériques avec les logiciels R, SAS et Splus*, Dunod, 2006.

[BAG 15] BAGOZZI B.E., "Forecasting civil conflict with zero-inflated count models", *Civil Wars*, vol. 17, no. 1, pp. 1–24, 2015.

[CAM 98] CAMERON A.C., TRIVEDI P.K., *Regression Analysis of Count Data*, Cambridge University Press, 1998.

[CAM 02] CAMPOLIETI M., "The recurrence of occupational injuries: estimates from a zero inflated count model", *Applied Economics Letters*, vol. 9, no. 9, pp. 595–600, 2002.

[CHA 12] CHARPENTIER A., DUTANG C., *L'actuariat avec R*, available at: https://cran.r-project.org/doc/contrib, 2012.

[CHE 11] CHEN X.-D., FU Y.-Z., "Model selection for zero-inflated regression with missing covariates", *Computational Statistics & Data Analysis*, vol. 55, no. 1, pp. 765–773, 2011.

[CON 92] CONSUL P.C., FAMOYE F., "Generalized Poisson regression model", *Communications in Statistics – Theory and Methods*, vol. 21, no. 1, pp. 89–109, 1992.

[COR 07] CORNILLON P.-A., MATZNER-LØBER E., *Régression : Théorie et applications*, Springer, 2007.

[CZA 05] CZADO C., MIN A., Consistency and asymptotic normality of the maximum likelihood estimator in a zero-inflated generalized Poisson regression, Report no. 423, Institut für Statistik der Ludwig-Maximilians-Universität München, 2005.

[CZA 07] CZADO C., ERHARDT V., MIN A. *et al.*, "Zero-inflated generalized Poisson models with regression effects on the mean, dispersion and zero-inflation level applied to patent outsourcing rates", *Statistical Modelling*, vol. 7, no. 2, pp. 125–153, 2007.

[DEB 97] DEB P., TRIVEDI P.K., "Demand for medical care by the elderly: a finite mixture approach", *Journal of Applied Econometrics*, vol. 12, no. 3, pp. 313–336, 1997.

[DEJ 08] DE JONG P., HELLER G.Z., *Generalized Linear Models for Insurance Data*, Cambridge University Press, 2008.

[DEM 77] DEMPSTER A.P., LAIRD N.M., RUBIN D.B., "Maximum likelihood from incomplete data via the EM algorithm", *Journal of the Royal Statistical Society, Series B*, vol. 39, no. 1, pp. 1–38, 1977.

[DEN 15] DENG D., ZHANG Y., "Score tests for both extra zeros and extra ones in binomial mixed regression models", *Communications in Statistics – Theory and Methods*, vol. 44, no. 14, pp. 2881–2897, 2015.

[DIA 17a] DIALLO A.O., DIOP A., DUPUY J.-F., "Asymptotic properties of the maximum-likelihood estimator in zero-inflated binomial regression", *Communications in Statistics – Theory and Methods*, vol. 46, no. 20, pp. 9930–9948, 2017.

[DIA 17b] DIALLO A.O., DIOP A., DUPUY J.-F., Estimation in zero-inflated binomial regression with missing covariates, available at: https://hal.archives-ouvertes.fr/hal-01585220/document, 2017.

[DIA 18] DIALLO A.O., DIOP A., DUPUY J.-F., "Analysis of multinomial counts with joint zero-inflation, with an application to health economics", *Journal of Statistical Planning and Inference*, vol. 194, pp. 85–105, 2018.

[DIO 11] DIOP A., DIOP A., DUPUY J.-F., "Maximum likelihood estimation in the logistic regression model with a cure fraction", *Electronic Journal of Statistics*, vol. 5, pp. 460–483, 2011.

[DIO 16] DIOP A., DIOP A., DUPUY J.-F., "Simulation-based inference in a zero-inflated Bernoulli regression model", *Communications in Statistics – Simulation and Computation*, vol. 45, no. 10, pp. 3597–3614, 2016.

[DOB 10] DOBSON A., *An Introduction to Generalized Linear Models*, 2nd ed., Taylor & Francis, 2010.

[DUP 17] DUPUY J.-F., "Inference in a generalized endpoint-inflated binomial regression model", *Statistics*, vol. 51, no. 4, pp. 888–903, 2017.

[EIC 66] EICKER F., "A multivariate central limit theorem for random linear vector forms", *The Annals of Mathematical Statistics*, vol. 37, no. 6, pp. 1825–1828, 1966.

[ERH 06] ERHARDT V., Verallgemeinerte Poisson und Nullenüberschuss-Regressionsmodelle mit regressiertem Erwartungswert, Dispersions- und Nullenüberschuss-Parameter und eine Anwendung zur Patentmodellierung, PhD thesis, Technische Universität München, 2006.

[FAH 85] FAHRMEIR L., KAUFMANN H., "Consistency and asymptotic normality of the maximum likelihood estimator in generalized linear models", *The Annals of Statistics*, vol. 13, no. 1, pp. 342–368, 1985.

[FAM 03] FAMOYE F., SINGH K.P., "On inflated generalized Poisson regression models", *Advances and Applications in Statistics*, vol. 3, no. 2, pp. 145–158, 2003.

[FAM 06] FAMOYE F., SINGH K.P., "Zero-inflated generalized Poisson model with an application to domestic violence data", *Journal of Data Science*, vol. 4, pp. 117–130, 2006.

[FAR 17a] FAROUGHI P., ISMAIL N., "Bivariate zero-inflated generalized Poisson regression model with flexible covariance", *Communications in Statistics – Theory and Methods*, vol. 46, no. 15, pp. 7769–7785, 2017.

[FAR 17b] FAROUGHI P., ISMAIL N., "Bivariate zero-inflated negative binomial regression model with applications", *Journal of Statistical Computation and Simulation*, vol. 87, no. 3, pp. 457–477, 2017.

[FEN 11] FENG J., ZHU Z., "Semiparametric analysis of longitudinal zero-inflated count data", *Journal of Multivariate Analysis*, vol. 102, no. 1, pp. 61–72, 2011.

[FRI 16] FRIENDLY M., MEYER D., ZEILEIS A., *Discrete Data Analysis with R: Visualization and Modeling Techniques for Categorical and Count Data*, CRC Press, Boca Raton, 2016.

[GIL 09] GILTHORPE M.S., FRYDENBERG M., CHENG Y. *et al.*, "Modelling count data with excessive zeros: the need for class prediction in zero-inflated models and the issue of data generation in choosing between zero-inflated and generic mixture models for dental caries data", *Statistics in Medicine*, vol. 28, no. 28, pp. 3539–3553, 2009.

[GOU 81] GOURIEROUX C., MONFORT A., "Asymptotic properties of the maximum likelihood estimator in dichotomous logit models", *Journal of Econometrics*, vol. 17, no. 1, pp. 83–97, 1981.

[GUP 04] GUPTA P.L., GUPTA R.C., TRIPATHI R.C., "Score test for zero inflated generalized Poisson regression model", *Communications in Statistics – Theory and Methods*, vol. 33, pp. 47–64, 2004.

[GUR 00] GURMU S., ELDER J., "Generalized bivariate count data regression models", *Economics Letters*, vol. 68, no. 1, pp. 31–36, 2000.

[GUY 01] GUYON X., *Statistique et Econométrie : Du modèle linéaire aux modèles non-linéaires*, Ellipses, 2001.

[HAL 00] HALL D.B., "Zero-inflated Poisson and binomial regression with random effects: A case study", *Biometrics*, vol. 56, pp. 1030–1039, 2000.

[HAL 04] HALL D.B., ZHANG Z., "Marginal models for zero inflated clustered data", *Statistical Modelling*, vol. 4, pp. 161–180, 2004.

[HE 10] HE X., XUE H., SHI N.-Z., "Sieve maximum likelihood estimation for doubly semiparametric zero-inflated Poisson models", *Journal of Multivariate Analysis*, vol. 101, no. 9, pp. 2026–2038, 2010.

[HE 15] HE H., WANG W., HU J. *et al.*, "Distribution-free inference of zero-inflated binomial data for longitudinal studies", *Journal of Applied Statistics*, vol. 42, no. 10, pp. 2203–2219, 2015.

[HEN 11] HENNINGSEN A., TOOMET O., "maxLik: A package for maximum likelihood estimation in R", *Computational Statistics*, vol. 26, no. 3, pp. 443–458, 2011.

[HIL 09] HILBE J., *Logistic Regression Models*, Taylor & Francis, 2009.

[HIL 11] HILBE J., *Negative Binomial Regression*, Cambridge University Press, 2011.

[HOS 00] HOSMER D.W., LEMESHOW S., *Applied Logistic Regression*, Wiley, 2000.

[JAC 15] JACKMAN S., pscl: Classes and methods for R developed in the political science computational laboratory, Stanford University, Stanford, California, 2015.

[JIA 10] JIANG J., *Large Sample Techniques for Statistics*, Springer, New York, 2010.

[JOH 05] JOHNSON N.L., KEMP A.W., KOTZ S., *Univariate Discrete Distributions*, Wiley, New York, 2005.

[KLE 08] KLEIBER C., ZEILEIS A., *Applied Econometrics with R*, Springer-Verlag, New York, 2008.

[LAM 92] LAMBERT D., "Zero-inflated Poisson regression, with an application to defects in manufacturing", *Technometrics*, vol. 34, no. 1, pp. 1–14, 1992.

[LAM 06] LAM K.F., XUE H., CHEUNG Y.B., "Semiparametric analysis of zero-inflated count data", *Technometrics*, vol. 62, no. 4, pp. 996–1003, 2006.

[LI 99] LI C.-S., LU J.-C., PARK J. *et al.*, "Multivariate zero-inflated Poisson models and their applications", *Technometrics*, vol. 41, no. 1, pp. 29–38, 1999.

[LI 12] LI C.-S., "Identifiability of zero-inflated Poisson models", *Brazilian Journal of Probability and Statistics*, vol. 26, no. 3, pp. 306–312, 2012.

[LIU 15] LIU Y., TIAN G.-L., "Type I multivariate zero-inflated Poisson distribution with applications", *Computational Statistics & Data Analysis*, vol. 83, pp. 200–222, 2015.

[LUK 16] LUKUSA T.M., LEE S.-M., LI C.-S., "Semiparametric estimation of a zero-inflated Poisson regression model with missing covariates", *Metrika*, vol. 79, no. 4, pp. 457–483, 2016.

[MAT 13] MATRANGA D., FIRENZE A., VULLO A., "Can Bayesian models play a role in dental caries epidemiology? Evidence from an application to the BELCAP data set", *Community Dentistry and Oral Epidemiology*, vol. 41, no. 5, pp. 473–480, 2013.

[MCC 89] MCCULLAGH P., NELDER J., *Generalized Linear Models*, 2nd ed., Chapman & Hall, 1989.

[MCL 08] MCLACHLAN G., KRISHNAN T., *The EM Algorithm and Extensions*, 2nd ed., Wiley, 2008.

[MON 80] MONFORT A., *Cours de probabilités*, Economica, 1980.

[MUL 86] MULLAHY J., "Specification and testing of some modified count data models", *Journal of Econometrics*, vol. 33, no. 3, pp. 341–365, 1986.

[NEL 72] NELDER J.A., WEDDERBURN R.W.M., "Generalized linear models", *Journal of the Royal Statistical Society, Series A (General)*, vol. 135, pp. 370–384, 1972.

[PIA 11] PIAZZA J.A., "Poverty, minority economic discrimination, and domestic terrorism", *Journal of Peace Research*, vol. 48, no. 3, pp. 339–353, 2011.

[PIZ 11] PIZER S.D., PRENTICE J.C., "Time is money: Outpatient waiting times and health insurance choices of elderly veterans in the United States", *Journal of Health Economics*, vol. 30, no. 4, pp. 626–636, 2011.

[PRA 09] PRASAD J.P., Zero-inflated Censored Regression Models: An Application with Episode of Care Data, available at: http://scholarsarchive.byu.edu/etd/2226, 2009.

[RCO 17] R CORE TEAM, R: A Language and Environment for Statistical Computing, R Foundation for Statistical Computing, Vienna, 2017.

[SAN 14] SANTIFORT-JORDAN C., SANDLER T., "An empirical study of suicide terrorism: A global analysis", *Southern Economic Journal*, vol. 80, no. 4, pp. 981–1001, 2014.

[SAR 06] SARMA S., SIMPSON W., "A microeconometric analysis of Canadian health care utilization", *Health Economics*, vol. 15, no. 3, pp. 219–239, 2006.

[SAR 09] SARI N., "Physical inactivity and its impact on healthcare utilization", *Health Economics*, vol. 18, no. 8, pp. 885–901, 2009.

[SOE 16] SOETAERT K., plot3D: Plotting Multi-Dimensional Data, 2016.

[STA 07] STASINOPOULOS D., RIGBY R., "Generalized additive models for location scale and shape (GAMLSS) in R", *Journal of Statistical Software*, vol. 23, no. 7, pp. 1–46, 2007.

[STA 13] STAUB K.E., WINKELMANN R., "Consistent estimation of zero-inflated count models", *Health Economics*, vol. 22, no. 6, pp. 673–686, 2013.

[STR 99] STREET A., JONES A., FURUTA A., "Cost-sharing and pharmaceutical utilisation and expenditure in Russia", *Journal of Health Economics*, vol. 18, no. 4, pp. 459–472, 1999.

[TIA 15] TIAN G.-L., MA H., ZHOU Y. *et al.*, "Generalized endpoint-inflated binomial model", *Computational Statistics & Data Analysis*, vol. 89, pp. 97–114, 2015.

[VAN 98] VAN DER VAART A., *Asymptotic Statistics*, Cambridge University Press, 1998.

[VAN 00] VAN IERSEL M.W., OETTING R.D., HALL D.B., "Imidacloprid applications by subirrigation for control of silverleaf whitefly (Homoptera: Aleyrodidae) on poinsettia", *Journal of Economic Entomology*, vol. 93, no. 3, pp. 813–819, 2000.

[VAS 09] VASECHKO O.A., GRUN-REHOMME M., BENLAGHA N., "Modélisation de la fréquence des sinistres en assurance automobile", *Bulletin Français d'Actuariat*, vol. 9, no. 18, pp. 41–63, 2009.

[VEN 02] VENABLES W.N., RIPLEY B.D., *Modern Applied Statistics with S*, 4th ed., Springer, New York, 2002.

[WAN 03] WANG P., "A bivariate zero-inflated negative binomial regression model for count data with excess zeros", *Economics Letters*, vol. 78, no. 3, pp. 373–378, 2003.

[WAN 17] WANG Y., Multivariate zero-inflated Poisson regression, Master's thesis, University of Minnesota Digital Conservancy, available at: http://hdl.handle.net/11299/189101, 2017.

[WED 74] WEDDERBURN R.W.M., "Quasi-likelihood functions, generalized linear models, and the Gauss–Newton method", *Biometrika*, vol. 61, pp. 439–447, 1974.

[WIN 13] WINKELMANN R., *Econometric Analysis of Count Data*, Springer, 2013.

[WOL 17] WOLODZKO T., extraDistr: Additional Univariate and Multivariate Distributions, R package version 1.8.5, 2017.

[XIA 07] XIANG L., LEE A.H., YAU K.K.W. *et al.*, "A score test for overdispersion in zero-inflated Poisson mixed regression model", *Statistics in Medicine*, vol. 26, no. 7, pp. 1608–1622, 2007.

[XIE 09] XIE F.-C., WEI B.-C., LIN J.-G., "Score tests for zero-inflated generalized Poisson mixed regression models", *Computational Statistics & Data Analysis*, vol. 53, no. 9, pp. 3478–3489, 2009.

[YAN 16] YANG M., DAS K., MAJUMDAR A., "Analysis of bivariate zero inflated count data with missing responses", *Journal of Multivariate Analysis*, vol. 148, pp. 73–82, 2016.

[YEE 16] YEE T.W., VGAM: Vector Generalized Linear and Additive Models, R package version 1.0-2, 2016.

[YEN 01] YEN S.T., TANG C.-H., SU S.-J.B., "Demand for traditional medicine in Taiwan: A mixed Gaussian Poisson model approach", *Health Economics*, vol. 10, no. 3, 2001.

[ZEI 02] ZEILEIS A., HOTHORN T., "Diagnostic checking in regression relationships", *R News*, vol. 2, no. 3, pp. 7–10, 2002.

[ZEI 04] ZEILEIS A., "Econometric computing with HC and HAC covariance matrix estimators", *Journal of Statistical Software*, vol. 11, no. 10, pp. 1–17, 2004.

[ZEI 06] ZEILEIS A., "Object-oriented computation of sandwich estimators", *Journal of Statistical Software*, vol. 16, no. 9, pp. 1–16, 2006.

[ZHU 17] ZHU H., LUO S., DESANTIS S.M., "Zero-inflated count models for longitudinal measurements with heterogeneous random effects", *Statistical Methods in Medical Research*, vol. 26, no. 4, pp. 1774–1786, 2017.

Index

Printed in the United States
By Bookmasters